Prittle, Prattle, Pain, Prayer, Praise Peace and Perfection

To:
Shelley
May you
have
many Blessings
Much Happiness
Continual Joy -
Nancy

MATTHEW 11:28 (29 & 30)
~~EPHES~~EPHESIANS 3:20
JEREMIAH 29: 11-13

ISBN-13: 978-0-9843647-7-4
ISBN-10 0-9846347-7-0

First printing, June 2012

Excerpts taken from other works listed in bibliography.

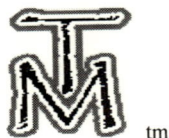

Published by:

ThomasMax Publishing
P.O. Box 250054
Atlanta, GA 30325
www.thomasmax.com

tm

Prittle, Prattle, Pain, Prayer, Praise, Peace and Perfection

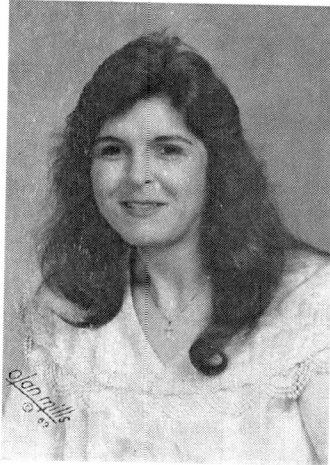

by Nancy Merritt Wiggins

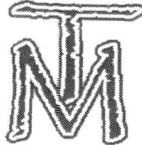

ThomasMax

Your Publisher
For The 21st Century

IN MY LIFE --

I HAVE HAD MUCH HAPPINESS -
      AND MUCH SADNESS --

I HAVE HAD MANY JOYS -
      AND MANY SORROWS --

ALWAYS FINDING -
   " GOD'S GRACE IS ALWAYS
      SUFFICIENT -
         IN LIFE
            AND
            IN DEATH" ---

With care
   and
      prayer
to each reader -
      Nancy

5033 WHEELER LAKE RD.
AUGUSTA, GA. 30909

(706) 854 · 0949

Nov. 4, 2014

Dear Shelley -

Thanks so much for all you do in serving our wonderful Lord and Savior.

There is no greater calling than praying for, working with and molding the hearts and lives of young people for God's guidance & His Glory. Just keep "loving them" all, even those that don't respond to being influenced now -- Just commit those to the Lord.

May God bless & strengthen you and those that work with you -

FOREWORDS

Sincerely,
Nancy

FOREWORD FROM THE AUTHOR

All of my life I had only wanted to be a wife and mother. In 2008, I found I was neither. My husband of 53 years died in February and my last surviving child died in May at age 41.

Since that time I have started the arduous journey of simply trying to find my new identity, seeking to find who I am, and what purpose my life has now. I have sought to handle my deep grief with God's help and with the many lessons and thoughts about life that I learned through the years from my daughter Melany.

This book is about Melany and the valiant way she handled her life after becoming disabled at twelve years of age.

Melany chose to be cheerful and spent her time caring for others. She believed that the most important things in life were: our personal relationship with Jesus Christ and our daily walk with HIM, our love and care for family, friends and mankind as a whole, and that our attitude about life keeps us kind and loving even when life is not kind.

This philosophy helped her rise above her constant pain and avoid becoming angry, bitter and resentful.

-- Nancy Merritt Wiggins

ADDITIONAL FOREWORDS

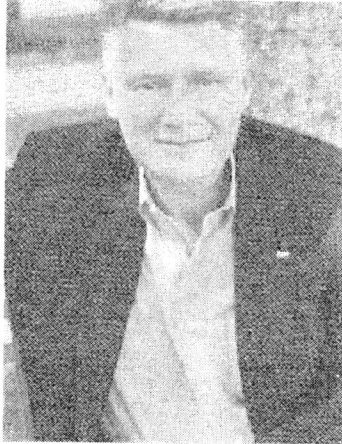

Dr. Mark E. Harris, Senior Pastor
First Baptist Church, Charlotte, NC
October 1, 2011

"The joy of the Lord is my strength." For some, that statement is a memory verse. For others, it has almost become a cliché. But for a young woman named Melany Wiggins, that verse, in my heart, was her life. The first time I met Melany was in a hospital room inside what was Saint Joseph's Hospital in Augusta, Georgia. A catheter to her heart, which had been placed to get critical medications to her body, was failing. As I approached her room that day, I had heard about Melany, and her battle with a disease that had left her body in a very debilitated an painful state. Her struggle with this disease was no doubt frustrating for Melany and the entire Wiggins family. Nothing could have prepared me for what I encountered that day, when this precious family stepped into my life.

The decision of the day centered on the fact that the line to Melany's heart needed to be replaced. A series of tests and a string of medical personnel coming in and out of her room had confirmed the situation. The doctor was very clear that the risks were immense. In fact, there was even a strong possibility Melany might not survive the procedure. During that visit, I came to see a young woman, her mom and dad, and her nephew, to be some of the most committed, determined, and faithful believers that I had ever encountered. They did not simply talk about faith. This family practiced faith. They did not simply talk about prayer. They really talked to the Lord Jesus. They did not simply speak of heaven. They knew it as a real place, where eternity is lived out by those who know Jesus as Savior. It was so obvious to me that these were not merely religious people, but that they were a people who had experienced a day by day relationship with the Living God. Decisions were made that day. Decisions would also be made in the future for Melany. I would always see a love, a trust, and a total dependence on God's plan. Whatever He wanted was fine with them.

In the pages that follow in this book you find testimonies and stories which will, without a doubt, touch your heart. In fact, in some places, you will even find yourself questioning if such responses to such crises are even possible. Let me just say, for over 5 years as the pastor of Curtis Baptist Church, and the Wiggins' pastor, I saw many of these trials. And yes, such responses are possible. But then again, the phrase "the joy of the Lord is my strength," was not cliché, nor simply a chorus, but it was a way of life for Melany and her family.

Today, Nancy Wiggins continues to live out her life, having buried her four children, and her dear husband James. She continues even now to exemplify the unusual peace that passes all understanding, just as her family did together. You will see, as the book unfolds, that they figured out what so many never understand: we are pilgrims passing through, strangers in this land; temporary in this earthly existence, remaining unattached to the things of this world. Why? Because we look forward to the day of no more sorrow, no more disease, no more pain, no more suffering, and no more night. Even so, Come Lord Jesus!

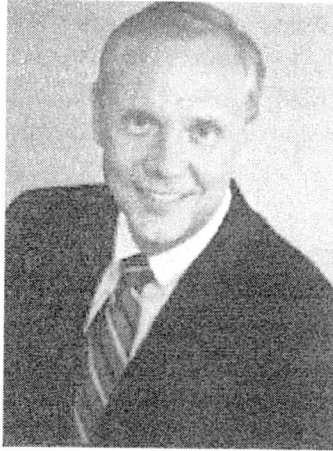

Dr. John Bryan
Georgia Baptist State Missionary
Atlanta, GA

There are some people you meet who leave little impression; they bounce off your life like two billiard balls which collide and go separate ways--acquaintances. Then there are those people who become important to you because they are valued to advance your work or they bring personal reward and even offer a helping hand up the next rung on life's ladder. These are the ones you treasure for a time, but when you separate, they move on and so do you--associates. However, there are some few individuals you encounter who leave indelible marks, because they are timeless in character and Christ-like in demeanor--inspirers. Melany Wiggins was the latter for me.

As her long-time pastor, I saw her literally grow up in stature, spirit and strength. Her illness became her platform for ministry, instead of a reason for complaint or pity. This made my multiple visits with Melany pleasurable, instead of painful, as she taught me life's lessons which she learned daily in her struggle to survive. The "pastor" became the "student" and many times I left her hospital room or home humbled in spirit and happy in heart, thanking God for a genuine encounter with Truth.

What would you do if you were stricken in the youth of life, unable to walk, continually reliant on others for daily help? Most curl up and hurl insults at God; few see it as an opportunity to prove His power. Melany's courage and unshakeable faith are a reflection of her earthly mom and dad, but more so, a mirror-image of her Heavenly Father.

The story line you will read in Nancy Wiggin's writings will bring you face-to-face with the reality that we each have a choice in life. We can choose to rebel against life's struggles wrought with pain or we can use every circumstance as an opportunity to advance God's purposes for ourselves and others. Melany chose to willfully follow Jesus' example of suffering as a privilege to share His love.

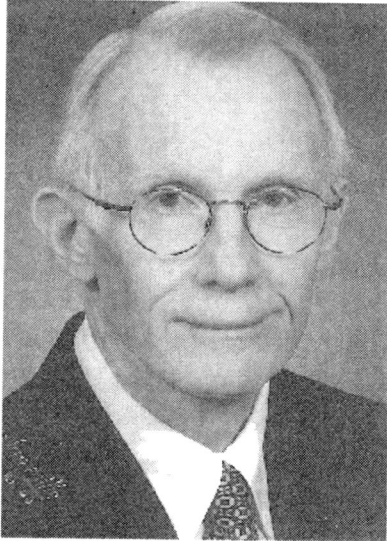

Dr. Richard Magruder, M.D.
Augusta, GA
August 17, 2011

I am pleased and honored to write a note of introduction for this book. Before my retirement in 2005, I was privileged to serve as Melany's primary care physician from the mid-1980's to retirement and as her dad, James', primary care physician for several years ending in 2005. Knowing Melany over this length of time, it was quite difficult and very frustrating to me to watch her gradual decline with such an elusive, complicated, and progressive disease. She was truly an inspiration to all who attended her.

I cannot recall her ever complaining about the care she received, the hours of waiting at her visits to multiple physicians, or our inability to make significant improvements in her physical being. She was a remarkably strong lady, mentally and spiritually. She was very determined, and was able to cope with her overwhelming health issues with remarkable grace and dignity. After reading this book, I believe you'll agree that Melany serves as a superb example of how one hopes to live out a very challenging and painful illness relying on her Christian faith to sustain her.

This narrative, however, includes not only Melany's story but that of her dad, James', ability to deal admirably with his final illness as well. It also tells of a family's ability to come together and cope with adversity over an extended period with a full measure of love, support, and unselfishness. In this age of broken, disturbed, and dysfunctional family relationships, it's reassuring to read of one family's togetherness in very trying circumstances. I do hope you will enjoy this read and take from it lessons we all should learn about family, faith, and how to deal most effectively with the most difficult of life's situations.

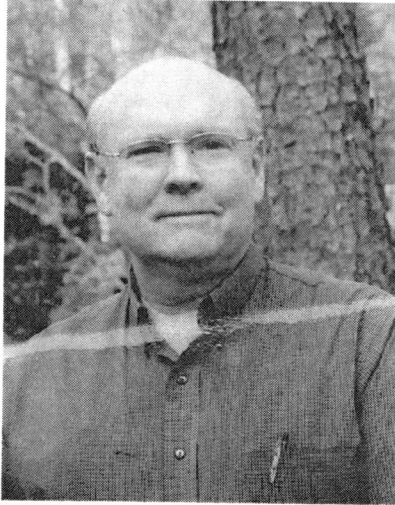

Dr. Dennis H. Jones, M.D.
Augusta, GA

It was my privilege to take care of Melany Wiggins for a number of years, until her death in 2008. The way she handled her illness was a wonderful testimony to her strong faith in Christ and His presence in her life. She radiated the grace of God in the worst of situations.

Her desire was to honor her Savior and show that tragedy from a human standpoint could be turned to triumph as she allowed Christ to reign in her life and express His presence through her.

If we could see her now, she would be radiant in her Lord's presence. She is now free from illness and pain, demonstrating as the scripture says, "Our present sufferings are not worth comparing to the glory that will be revealed in us." Romans 8:18.

May her life be an encouragement to others as it has been to me.

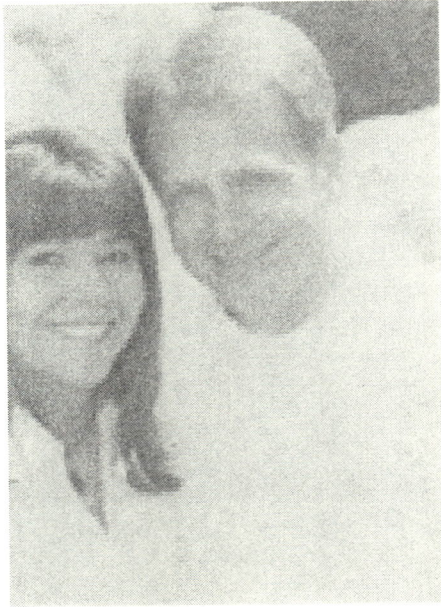

Dr. Mark Sterling (with wife Michelle)
Senior Pastor
Curtis Baptist Church
Augusta, GA

Mark's Foreword:

Melany Wiggins' journey through life with Behcet's Disease is a story of life, love and God. Melany's story is a wakeup call to value life to the fullest every day. It reveals insights needed to face unexpected challenges in life and inspires the human spirit to never give up but always trust God with everything. It is real, honest, and enlightening on how to depend on God when traveling through seasons of darkness and contains nuggets of wisdom for living no matter one's age or station in life.

One of Melany's college professors, who was a professing agnostic noted, "Melany is the only person I've ever met that inspired me to want to really know a more about Jesus Christ."

I pray Melany's story will do the same for you. May God bless and challenge you as you read and reflect on Melany's journey.

Michelle's Foreword:

James 1:2 says, "Consider it pure joy, my brothers whenever you face trials of many kinds."

This verse describes Nancy Wiggins' life! She has been an example to me from the day I first encountered her. She is full of God's joy and truly has counted it all joy as she has faced many trials both large and small. Her radiant face always reflects the joy of the Lord and her love and care of others. Anyone who reads this story will be encouraged that God really can bring joy in all things!

Rev. Sherrill Dunn,
Associate Pastor
Curtis Baptist Church
Augusta, GA

Melany Wiggins was more than just a name. She was an awesome treasure in an earthen vessel dedicated to the glory of God. The tent in which she lived was tattered and torn by a lifelong disease, but her inner person was a testimony to the power of God.

When I think of Melany, I am reminded of the words that the apostle Paul wrote to the Corinthian church: "...we are afflicted in every way, but not crushed, perplexed but not despairing, persecuted but not forsaken, struck down but not destroyed, ...so that the life of Jesus may also be manifested in our body." However, as for Melany, she never felt persecuted. Yes, the body was weak, but the inner person was becoming stronger by the day. She had as strong a spirit as any person I have ever known: Invincible, unshakable, stouthearted, courageous.

More than anything that can be said about Melany is that she loved the Lord Jesus Christ with all her heart. She could always find a way to encourage someone; her pain never hindered her missionary spirit. She was an encourager to hurting people. She was not one to complain about her struggles, but always ready to walk with anyone through theirs. Melany lived out II Corinthians 1:3-4 every day of her life. She used every opportunity to share God's love in word and deed and to share another's burden. She was always ready to comfort those who were suffering with the same comfort that she had received from God.

Someone might ask, "What was her secret? How could she always have joy and a positive outlook on life?" It is no secret. The key to her attitude was an absolute surrender of her total being to the Lord Jesus Christ. She had been bought with a price and she was Christ's vessel. She trusted Him, accepted His will and used what God gave her to His glory. The words recorded in I Corinthians 10:31 remind me of Melany Wiggins: "Whether, then you eat or drink or whatever you do, do all to the glory of God."

Dr. Bucky Kennedy
Senior Pastor
First Baptist Church
Vidalia, GA

I first met Melany at Georgia Southern College through the ministry of Fellowship of Christian Athletes, a Christian organization in which we were both active.

Melany had an incredible smile and infectious laugh which is incredible given her circumstances; Behcet's Disease had crippled her body but not her heart. She got around in a wheelchair and never desired to be anything but encouraging. If she was in pain, and most days she was, one would never know it by her attitude and determination to live life according to her faith and not her feelings.

It has been said that adversity reveals character but Melany's adversity revealed Christ. Although she would need assistance from others from time to time, she desired most to be a servant to others. Her independence was born not of pride, that she might prove others wrong, but that she might prove Christ as her sufficiency. She wasn't stubborn; she was content to fight with a holy determination.

Melany encouraged me to be a better Christian; to purpose my faith to dictate to my circumstances instead of my circumstances to dictate to my faith.

COMMENTS

My grandmother is without a doubt the spiritually-strongest person that I have ever had the pleasure to know, she truly walks by faith. Melany was the supreme example of how to face and, in many ways, overcome adversity. My grandfather was the standard of how to be a morally rich man, while maintaining a firm, but most kind-hearted disposition. It has been a pleasure to live with, and later, near them my entire life, though the circumstances that brought us together often were not. May every reader glimpse the people I knew and loved while enjoying their story, but also digesting its true contents -- The Glory Of GOD.

Jake Wiggins, Augusta, GA

* * * * *

Phil. 4:13: I can do all things through Christ who strengthens me. So True! That is the verse Mel wrote in the Bible that she special ordered for my 40th Birthday 11 years ago! She knew my eyes had changed with my new age and was so sweet to get me the much needed large print to help me out! That is what my wonderful friend Mel always did for me and anyone that knew her, she always was there to help us out. Through her, Christ's light shined and was always on and never faded, even when my sweet friend's body was oh , so fading.

From her room my sister in Christ knew more then most of us will ever know about life here on Earth. Mel and I talked on the phone for hours at a time, late night was our time! We did this several times a week for many years and I could ask her about anything and I mean anything. She never had to say wait a minute let me Google that, she always knew the right answer. I know with all my Heart my friend is in the arms of Jesus and I look forward to our talks again when Jesus calls me home. For now I still find myself going to the phone to call her, almost every week.

I am truly grateful that my awesome sister Julie shared her wonderful College friend with me and I am so thankful to Christ for letting His Angel Girl Bless all whom came in contact with her. My human self cannot say the words to describe Melany, Mel, Mimi Wiggins and how much she is loved and missed!

So I will say as Mrs. Wiggins always said to both of us while we were still talking on the phone, when she was on her way to bed. Something she & Mel had said to each other every night, since Mel was two- (I have always said this since the first time I heard her say it)--

" I Luv ou and Dod Bess you wittle hart!"

Amy Fox, Orlando, FL

* * * * *

If my memory serves me right, I first met M.W. (Melany Wiggins) in 1979 when she was ~12 years old and I was ~20 years old. She was a student at Curtis Baptist School and I was a part of a leadership discipleship group(led by Tom Lowry) that was encouraged to go to the upper school at lunch to spend time with and get to know the students. I'll never forget her smile and the way she 'humored me' as I awkwardly tried to make conversation with her and the other students. The day I met her she was walking with the assistance of special crutches. Throughout her junior high and high school years she went back and forth from the crutches to a wheelchair and eventually was in the wheelchair full time by the time she reached college. The ~30 years of our friendship (which started at CBS that day at lunch) I watched her go from crutches, to a wheelchair, and eventually to being pretty much bed bound. She never lost her focus (loving Jesus and loving others), or her sense of humor. She went on youth trips, excelled in her studies at CBS, and went away to college. Each milestone amazed us all. Though she couldn't 'physically' participate fully in many activities, she wanted to be a part and was there for us emotionally and spiritually. I look forward to reading this book that her mama, Nancy, has been working on so lovingly and diligently all these years.

April Greene Lowry, North Augusta, SC

* * * * *

Thousands of students have crossed my life-path in the 43 years I've been involved in the education business. Most of them are just a blur in my memory. Once in awhile, a student makes an indelible impression. Melany Wiggins was one of those who made that life-time memory. I remember the first time I met Melany. It was after church on a Sunday morning when she was just a little girl. I was the Headmaster of Curtis Baptist School and Melany was a pre-schooler, darting around the parking lot speaking to everyone and exploring everything. She was always a joy to have in school. Her fun-loving spirit and great attitude made her everyone's favorite. It wasn't long until health problems raised their ugly heads. Her attitude was getting a severe test. The great thing about it was that she always passed the test! An illustration of this came one spring break about the time Melany was completing elementary school. The school had planned a trip and chartered a bus to Disney World for all students who wanted to go. Melany wanted very much to go, but her mother doubted that she had the stamina for an arduous trip. Nancy discussed it with my wife and me. We volunteered to be her special chaperones, and she was to stick close to us at all times. Melany had a great time. We contacted the first aid station at Disney, and they provided a space with a cot so Melany could take frequent breaks. This was the kind of spirit that enabled Melany to succeed in spite of life-long bad health. She wasn't about to let not feeling good stop her. Oh, and did I say Mr. and Mrs. Holt had a great time at Disney, too?! Just being with Melany was always a lift to the spirit.

Arvil E. Holt, Blythe, Georgia
Former Headmaster, Curtis Baptist School, Augusta, Georgia

* * * * *

You may not choose to use my "testiment of devotion" in your book. But as I was so impressed with Melany's honesty, I would be doing her memory a disservice if I weren't honest also.

Since I was Melany's Counselor and friend throughout her years at Georgia Southern and just a 'friend' in the years following her graduation, my memories are very different in some ways than any of the other testimonials. I continued to visit with Melany after she graduated and up until a few months prior to her death.

I would offer a resounding "AMEN!" to all the above beautiful and meaningful expressions of Melany's life and how she fought the good and great fight to the end, always telling of God's love for all of us, always surrendering to His love.

However, as her Counselor there were many, many secrets, *dark* secrets that she shared with me that truly broke my heart to hear. It is unbelievable what she suffered (beyond her illness) ! Unbelievable! But Melany was always honest to the core of her being, wasn't she?   There were those who should have begged her forgiveness...but didn't. But she forgave them without ever letting them know that she did. She taught me so much about courage, strength, endurance, kindness, friendship and loving....in spite of! But most of all....Forgiveness!!

Thoughtfully submitted,

Audrey Campbell (Retired)
Licensed Professional Counselor, LPC
111 Elliswood Drive, Statesboro,GA

* * * * *

Mel was truly one of God's angels here on earth. She had joy in all circumstances and I never heard her wish her life had been any different. She shared the Lord with all around her because of the joy He had put in her heart was obvious to all. I am blessed to have known and cared for her. I thank God for bringing her into my life.

Brenda Wilson, RN, North Augusta, S.C.

* * * * *

I met Melany in 1987 when I started dating and eventually married her brother Ric. We had a son we named Jake and he was the light of her life it seemed. Sometimes I think that is why she held on as long as she did.

Melany was already in a wheelchair when we met and I watched her go through more pain and suffering than I thought any person could ever take. But she told me one time that God had a plan for her and if the life she had of pain and suffering was His plan then it must be for a good reason. She never wavered in her faith of her God. Even her last words reflect that. They were: "I see Jesus." And then she was gone to us until we meet her again in heaven. She has always been my inspiration and always will be. She touched my life in ways that she never knew. Whenever I think things are bad I just think of Melany and know that no matter what my problems are at the time they could always be worse. She is a light that still shines in my heart to this day and for all the rest of my days.

Charlotte Wiggins Bonifay, FL Melany's sister-in-love

* * * * *

Melany was the most beautiful spirited person I have ever met. God used her to touch so many people and He has used your family as an inspiration to many--I'm one of them.

Thank you for sharing your family with others.

May God give you His peace and strength to carry on.

Faye Wright, North Augusta, S.C.

* * * * *

Words will never be able to express the special place Melany has in my heart. The Wiggins family is like no other I've ever been blessed to know.

I so admire how you live your faith every day.

I will miss Melany forever!

Gayle Virgo RN, North Augusta, S.C.

* * * * *

A TRIBUTE TO MELANY WIGGINS
(A Godly student I shall never forget!)

When the Lord pulls back the curtain
　Of precious memories;
When He allows a backward glance
　At things held dear to me--
When His camera brings in focus
　Lives that bless continually---
I SEE YOU.

When I think of straight "A" students
　(Making "A's" in spite of pain.)
Setting goals that seemed unreachable--
　Adding new ones when attained;
When I think of Valedictorians
　(The best to claim that fame)
I SEE YOU.

When I think of scary moments,
　Or of silly, impish grins,
Or times when girl and teacher
　Talked together friend to friend,
When I think of inspiration,
　(Courage--faith--without an end);
I SEE YOU

Curtis School became the richer,
　Every teacher grew more wise
As you helped us see the future

Shining through your trusting eyes!
I THANK YOU!

A grateful teacher, Geraldine F. Holt, Blythe, GA, January 30, 1986

* * * * *

Have you ever been touched by an angel?--I have--let me tell you about it.

Her name was Melany Wiggins and she touched so many people. Melany wanted to serve as a missionary but because of her serious illness, she could not go. I was called to go to East Asia to tell the Good News. Melany was my #1 prayer partner. When I would return home for a couple of months, the first place I would go was to see Melany. You see she was my partner and I feel what happened in Asia was to her account. I would go to see her to bring her encouragement. However, I always left there walking on air, because as I said, I was touched by an angel. All of you will one day see and touch this angel if you are right with our Lord.

Joye Neal, Augusta, GA

* * * * *

Melany and I met in the Fall of 1985 at Georgia Southern College and became close friends quite quickly! Then again how could I not become close friends with someone who walks up to me at the Library a week or so after we had met and tells me that I have to give her a shot because her life depended on it and she couldn't give it to herself. And although she knew I had never given anyone a shot before in my life she trusted me enough to ask me to help her. Yes, that was the beginning of a friendship that would change my life forever.

Melany and I would talk for hours and hours at a time and never run out of things to say - we talked about our faith, our hopes, our dreams, our struggles, our fears, and our relationships. We laughed together, we cried together and we stood in the gap in prayer for each other. And throughout the years despite anything going on in her life she was always ready and willing to listen, pray, offer advice, and/or be an encourager anytime I needed her.

One of our other favorite things to do together was going to the beach! We loved to look for shells, go crabbing or fishing or watch the sun set. It seemed that almost everytime that Mel and I watched the sunset, God would show up and paint the sky in some of the most amazing colors just for us because He knew how much we admired His handiwork. As I look back over the past 20 years I know that God put Melany in my life for many reasons.

Melany is probably one of the most patient, loving, caring, thoughtful, tolerant, people I have ever known. She was wise beyond her years and always knew the right thing to say no matter what the circumstance. Although she lived in a tremendous amount of physical pain, she never complained or gave up. Melany chose to look at every day as a gift and live it out for the Lord!

Love and miss you my friend!

Julie Edwards, Brunswick, Georgia

* * * * *

How can I possibly condense into one or two paragraphs the impact Melany has had on my life? I have known and loved her since she was a child as her mother is one of my dearest friends. I saw and marveled at her indomitable spirit during all those years of her illness. I prayed for her and cried with her. Many,many times I went to encourage her in her worse times, and I ended up being the one encouraged. I saw her in some of the most pain-wracked moments of her life, and not once did I go away without a time of shared laughter. She suffered most of her short life. Yet she brought so much happiness to so many people that my memory of her is of joy. I used (and am still using) her as an example so many times that my family and friends, though they never met her, know her.

I'd like to share just one experience we had together. She trained for and participated in our Acteens Activators mission trip to Kansas City. Although she was already on crutches by the time we went, she was determined to go and do her part in the Vacation Bible School we held in a small church. She worked with the babies. She could not carry the babies and hold on to her crutches, so she laid down her crutches and sat on the floor with the 'crawlers'. Some careless person left the door to the nursery ajar and one baby crawled out. Melany crawled after and caught the baby and got it back in the nursery. When the session was over, we found Melany in the floor surrounded by perfectly happy babies. She rarely ever let her handicaps prevent her from doing anything she set her heart on doing.

She was at the same time my best friend, my shining example, and the daughter I never had.

Margaret Brown, Laurens, SC

* * * * *

My earliest childhood memories are of Melany. We were inseparable and closer than most sisters. Even in preschool we were there for each other. We shared birthdays, Christmas', and most days together. We rode bikes, climbed trees and played at the creek for many hours. As we grew older and her medical problems worsened I helped care for her and witnessed the increasing pain and suffering she had to endure. Through it all she remained positive and kept her caring attitude toward others. I married and moved away but distance didn't change our friendship. I feel truly blessed to have been her best friend. My life is richer for the experience. I miss you Melany.

Mary Faulk Mills, Statesville, NC

* * * * *

Melany was a sweet, kind, generous person. She really never complained!   She was always nice to "her nurses" Not one of us ever minded taking care of Melany. She was always a Joy!

Mrs. Wiggins you were so wonderful with her. You gave all you could give!! You were a wonderful mother!

Maxine Washington RN, and Nurses Teresa Beman, Sondra Ward and Debbie Greshan, Augusta, GA

* * * * *

I cannot remember the exact time I met Melany, but I do remember her chasing my brother (Kevin) around the tree when they were in kindergarten. Melany was always full of determination, joy and happiness.   I have many special memories of her. We did Acteens together and when she could we shared youth trips. I remember one trip we went on when she said she was going even if she had to come home in a box. I was scared that whole week that she would not make it. Through all of her pain and struggles I never saw Melany complain. She stayed strong in her faith.

My funniest memory of Melany happened at the hospital. I stayed with her one night so her mom could go home and rest. When the nurse came in she thought I was Melany and got upset trying to figure out how she got out of bed and into the chair where her mom usually slept.

Melany was determined to go away to college and graduate. One night she wasn't doing well and her mom needed someone to ride with her to Georgia Southern I can honestly say I have never ridden that fast before.   I was thankful we didn't get stopped for speeding, but I was more thankful we made it there alive. I don't think I have ever seen Mrs. Wiggins move that fast.

Melany will always have a special place in my heart.   She taught me how to be thankful for little things and no matter what the circumstances are to never give up. She was a special blessing that I will always cherish.

Missing You,

Rhonda Vaughn Hazle, Gaffney, South Carolina

* * * * *

To My Sweet Melany,

What a beautiful angel butterfly! I thank my blessed Lord for allowing us to praise Him together! I will always remember our Bible Studies and prayer time together! Thanks for always listening to me and giving me such wonderful guidance and wisdom. You always amazed me for the great counseling you gave me and everyone around you.

Thanks for encouraging me to be the child of God that He created me to be! Thanks for always looking at the positive side of everything!

Love, Runy

Veronica Runette Whitaker, Augusta, Georgia

* * * * *

I had the privilege of being one of Melany's physical therapists, first when she was recovering from knee surgery at St. Joseph's Hospital, later when she was an outpatient, and then when she was a home health patient, over the span of several years.

One of my strongest impressions of Melany was of her incredible courage and faith. She was a sweet, generous, and loving friend, while coping with a cruel and painful illness.

I will never forget her smile.

Sally Wright, PT, Augusta, Georgia

* * * * *

I didn't get to know Melany as a close friend until later in life, in spite of us both attending the same school in the same time frame (she was Class of '85; I was Class of '83). I initially started visiting her, showing her my photos and telling her about my travels, in the hopes of cheering her up and taking her mind off the pain she frequently endured. While I may have been partially successful in doing so, I probably walked away with the greater blessing from our time together. She introduced me to her beloved St. Simons Island, and I was privileged to spend much time there with the Wiggins Family, and I still make trips there, missing Melany very much every time. She had a way of making everything fun!

Whether it was her entertaining me with the latest exploits of the Wiggins Family or helping me work through some issue of my own, she was more interested in helping others, not focusing on herself. That servant attitude was just one of the ways that you could see Christ through Melany.

Stan Brassell, Augusta, GA

* * * * *

Melany was a true inspiration for people, it was a true pleasure to fly her down and back from St. Simons. I would have gladly done it several times a year. What a really delightful person to be around, and as I said to her dad at the airport when he wanted to promise anything I ever needed, She'd already given it to me. God Bless You.

Steve Thompson, Evans, GA, Melany's last pilot

* * * * *

I've always regarded Melany as the most inspirational and accomplished person that I've ever had the pleasure to know. I always looked forward to her smiling face and talking with her

at the Turk family reunion at Chestnut Mountain. Just like James & Ric she will truly be missed.
God bless her soul and your heart.

Mike Ferguson, Gainesville, GA (cousin)

* * * * *

What a joy it was to know Melany and grow up with her. Even in her lowest moments she could always make me laugh. So many, many great memories.

Tony Hathaway, North Augusta, S.C., friend since birth

* * * * *

How fortunate we all are to have had Mel in our lives! I remember so many Christmases shared with her at St. Joseph's. There were so many good memories.. she always was the ultimate for smiling in adversity. She taught me SO much about life.

Esther Hicks, RN, North Augusta, S.C.

* * * * *

There is no way I can fully express what the Wiggins family has meant to me over the past 25 years. Melany was a beloved sister in the Lord and a constant encourager with her love for Jesus Christ and her wisdom.

Robert Eubanks, Ft.. Worth, TX

* * * * *

Nancy, May God bless you for the wonderful example that you have been to each of us over the years, showing us what it truly means to love and care for those that God brings into our lives. You have amazed me since Ric & I were in 5th. Grade. I know without a doubt that you continue to allow God to be glorified in all things! We will keep you in our prayers, while thanking God for such a faithful servant!

Kathy Jones, Lavonia, GA

* * * * *

In the entire time that I knew Melanie she was without a doubt the most positive and loving person in all of her endeavors regardless of her problems. In her life she made lemonade out of lemons and never complained about her life. She loved life , her friends, her lord and her family. I always said that when I grew up I wanted to be like Melanie. I loved her with all my heart and appreciate the opportunity of knowing her and her family.

Janice Petsch R.N., Evans, GA

* * * * *

To know her was to love her- it's a phrase you often hear, but quite rare for this simple statement to fit someone as easily & absolutely as it fit Melany throughout her life.

I met Melany in kindergarten & she energetically filled her childhood, and by default, all those around her, with a constant whirlwind of motion, laughter, learning, adventure and on occasion, "foot down, hands-on-her hips" kind of stubborn. As time went by, it became clear what an important role those attributes would play in her life.

Melany had an extraordinary capacity to love and she related to people with such patience & ease. During one of our marathon phone calls, we talked about the pain & difficulty I was having following surgery. She was so empathetic, understanding & re-assuring. I asked her something I'd often wondered- with all the terrible pain and frightening situations she'd faced over the years, how could she have so much genuine compassion, as this was surely miniscule in comparison? She told me the worst pain she'd experienced in her life was no different than the worst pain I'd ever experienced in mine, that it was all relative to what each of us had been through. Melany wasn't perfect, she made mistakes & she didn't pretend that life was always wonderful or fair, but she was blessed with a strong and wonderful family, as well as this remarkable way of embracing life's challenges with such a positive attitude, they became gifts that could be used to inspire others.

I'm forever grateful that God blessed me with Melany's friendship.

Nancy Maxwell Shealy, Evans, GA

* * * * *

Some things I remember about my friend Melany:

Our families went to Ridgecrest, N.C. during music week each year. We enjoyed the Day Camp, Rexcreation Area, Nibble Nook Ice Cream Parlor, throwing rocks & walks in the creek, and just hanging out and having fun. If you knew Melany back then, she was always in gear and ready to go.

On one trip, my brother Greg and I were climbing a tree when one of the branches broke. Greg fell to the ground, with the branch still in his hand. Melany was right there with us. I'm sure she was the one who ran for help. These trips were just one of the many times I remember spending with Melany. We loved to sing, play and just have fun.

I especially remember Melany's love for God, for her friends, family and others. You could see the light of Christ shine through her. She never gave me a hard time, or judged me, but I knew she prayed for me.

The most important thing I remember was her love and her friendship for me in spite of my short comings. In my opinion she was wise, and strong and had more peace than anyone I ever knew.

Doug Barton, Jr., Grovetown, Georgia

* * * * *

Melany Wiggins--

Our friendship...time spent as if it were today standing still; words spoken, still ringing true in my mind. Laughter, joking, listening and sharing "the simple", and "the not so simple . . . confidences of friendship. Being there in the little and the big situations that arose in both our lives. No judgement towards each other was and still is a "Blessed Friendship."

What makes a true friendship as ours, and so many to ring so true? "A true friend loves at all times" (KJV), and Melany was that type of friend to all of those around her. A constant and steadfast friend.

Tracey Barton, Grovetown, GA

Lovingly dedicated to:

The Glory of God

My grandson Jake Wiggins--
for continuing love, help, and
care for James, Melany, & myself

Dr. Richard Magruder--
for many hours spent helping
with the manuscript and for many years
of caring for our family and others.

CHAPTER LISTINGS

*THE SCRIPTURES, POEMS AND COMMENTS were
selected with great care and prayer for the proper chapters.
Hopefully they will perhaps touch a Heart or
Life that needs to receive their message.*

CHAPTER I
PRITTLE

*"HE MAKETH THE BARREN WOMAN TO KEEP HOUSE,
AND TO BE A JOYFUL MOTHER OF CHILDREN. PRAISE YE
THE LORD." Psalm 113:9*

*"A MERRY HEART MAKETH A CHEERFUL
COUNTENANCE."
Proverbs 15:13a*

After the heartache of being unable to have a child for several years, the Lord blessed our home with a precious baby boy on March 20, 1960.

James and I had worked hard, purchased our first home and our life was just wonderful, though I had only carried our first baby for six months and we had lost one young child. Many of our friends had started their families. We observed the things they did right and the things that could be improved in raising and nurturing children.

Ric, our firstborn was a perfect joy. He was sweet, kind and obedient. Occasionally he had to be reprimanded as all children do but he responded well to discipline. We often reminded him of how much he was loved, and that we wanted other people to love and enjoy him as well.

We felt we had just the right balance and amount of needed correction with lots of love and encouragement in our family. Thus, we were rearing a happy, well-adjusted child that was a joy to everyone.

Around the age of five Ric started praying for a baby brother and wanted to name him Will. Two years later, to the delight of everyone and the surprise of my doctors, we found out that we were having another baby.

When I carried Ric he was a very calm, sedate baby. He moved so seldom that we laughingly called him lazy. Early on I knew that this baby was very different. She was perpetual motion. She started moving early and never slowed down. She constantly jumped, kicked and wiggled. She kicked so hard she bruised my ribs and caused me great pain. It was as if she could not wait to get out and start enjoying life.

We had season tickets to our local high school football games. I told my obstetrician, "Before the band could be seen and heard in the distance as it came onto the field at halftime that she would start jumping and flipping." Dr. Goldberg and his wife had seats two rows above us. He had asked me to let him know when she started doing this. At the next game James motioned to them that the commotion had started. He and his wife came down to feel the activity. He was so amazed that he summoned two other doctor friends to come and feel the movement. We could barely hear the drums in the band but the baby was well aware of the vibrations.

We became a weekly spectacle as those around us joined in to feel the baby leaping and jumping as long as the band played. She always loved music and had great rhythm.

I have often wondered, although I really do not believe, that we were smug in our efforts involving the rearing of our children. We were just very thankful for our first child and his responding to discipline as he did. Both children brought much joy in different ways to us, our family and to others.

I thanked God many times we had never verbally criticized any of our friends or other parents for the way their children acted. For years later many of our friends expressed delight that we had been blessed with a second child that apparently had never read the child-rearing manuals and books and could care less that we had.

Finally on January 30, 1967, our home was blessed with a beautiful delightful daughter. We were so very thankful to have a healthy baby girl who was just perfect.

Melany was born at 10:30 a.m. Her daddy went to Ric's

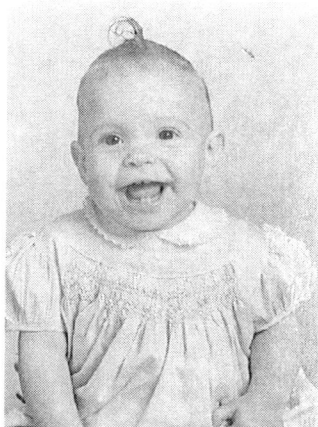

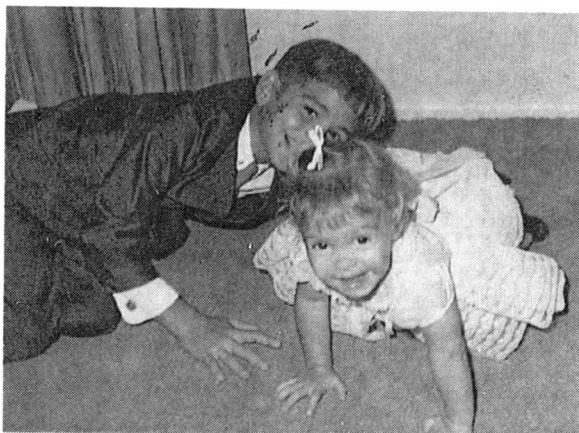

Melany, at right with Ric, below in basinet, bottom in crib

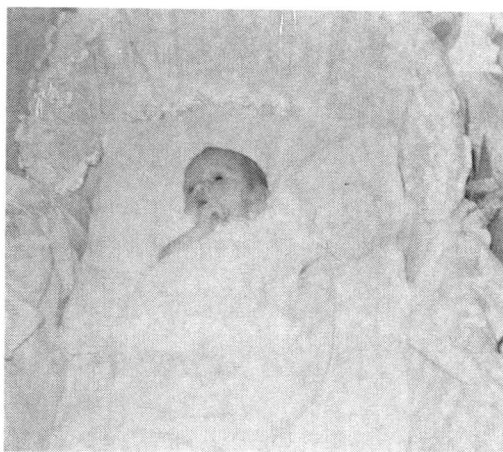

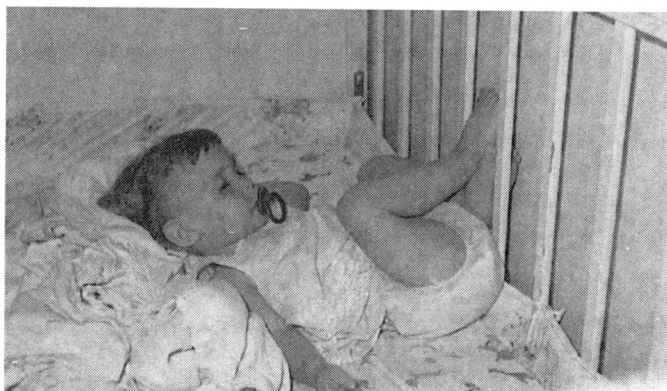

school, he was in the first grade, to tell him about the baby. The children were lining up to go to lunch. Ric ran to his dad because he knew I was in the hospital and the baby was coming. James told him he had a little sister named Melany, a name that he had helped pick out "just in case" it was a girl. His countenance fell and he dropped his little head as he walked off. He turned back and lamented, "This is so embarrassing, I told them that I was getting a brother named Will."

As indicated by the titles of these chapters this child gave new meaning to Dr. Dobson's book, *The Strong-Willed Child*, which I often read and referred to. She came into this world feeling she was in charge of everything. James once compared us to persons holding a tiger by the tail. You knew you could not really control her. All you could do was hang on and try to enjoy the ride. It seemed she was determined from the beginning to have her own way regardless, and I was just as determined she wouldn't.

In Florence Littauer's book *Personality Plus*, she lists the different personalities. She describes the choleric personality as one who at an early age looks through the bars of their crib wondering when not if, they will be taking over the world.

I wished many times that our loving Heavenly Father (who must have a real sense of humor) had reminded me He had given this child such a strong will and determination so she would not be defeated by the many difficulties and battles she must fight and endure all of her life. I don't know what we would have done differently as parents if we had known. We felt then as we do now years later that all children, especially strong-willed ones, and even disabled ones need structure, discipline and a lot of love and laughter in their lives.

Ric loved his baby sister dearly and enjoyed watching her grow. In the spring he and his friend David (the youngest of three brothers), were playing on the back screened-in porch while I was in the kitchen cooking supper.

David asked, "Did that baby really come out of your mother's tummy?" Ric answered, "No, I'll tell you how she got here if you won't tell anybody." This surprised me. We had explained to him according to his questions and his understanding, all about how babies were born and how they were planted by God at the time of conception. We told him this was very special to families and he should not discuss it with his friends because their parents would want to share it with them when they felt they were old enough to understand. Ric usually did as we asked. I listened intently as he told the following story to David.

"David, you have been to St. Joseph's hospital, right?"

David nodded.

"Well my Mama and Daddy prayed and ordered a baby from heaven. When God got it made He called Dr. Goldberg. Dr. Goldberg called my mama at five o'clock in the morning and said, 'The baby is coming.'"

My Daddy took me to your house and he took my mama to the hospital. They waited there until 10:30 when a special angel no one could see dropped the baby into the big basket on top of the hospital. The doctor went up and got her and brought her to my mama and daddy."

David inquired, "What happens if the babies miss the basket?"

Ric quickly replied, "Haven't you seen the baby graves at the cemetery? They missed the basket and splattered on the roof."

David was also seven years old but he just couldn't grasp all of this. He asked, "Is this what your mama and daddy told you?"

Ric hesitated and replied thoughtfully, "No, David, you would never believe what they told me. And I don't either."

On Mother's Day our church had a baby dedication service and with thanksgiving in our hearts we dedicated Melany to our Lord. Today we are thankful for everyday we had with her. Although some have been very trying we have had much joy and lots of fun.

We realized from the very beginning this baby had a very different personality. When she wanted to eat she didn't just cry; she screamed until my milk, the bottle, or her cereal (in 1967 the pediatricians started cereal at four weeks) satisfied her. Then she was very happy until the next feeding which, even if we tried moving it up was to no avail. She still screamed until she was ready to stop. She did not have the different pitches of fussing or crying like other babies. Her volume was wide open loud every time.

Ric enjoyed holding her, feeding her (when she stopped screaming), and helping to bathe her. We had a bassinette (hardly ever heard of these days) we had used with him as a baby. Every morning I set it up in the kitchen and placed her in the little hammock-type support. The lower part of the support lowered down into the bottom and kept the head and upper part of the body out of the water. Melany never liked a bath, probably because she wasn't in control of the situation.

One morning as Ric was helping me bathe her, the hammock support broke apparently from fatigue because we had let everyone use the bassinette during the seven years since our last baby. I immediately retrieved her from the water which had covered her head and body. I rinsed her off, wrapped her in a warm towel, then snuggled and attempted to comfort her.

An hour later she was still screaming loudly. I called our pediatrician to see if he would check her to be sure that she was alright. Ric and I took her in the car to the doctor. Normally riding settled her down but not today! She was still bellowing loudly when we arrived. The doctor checked her eyes to be sure they had not been irritated by the tearless soap. He checked her ears and listened to her chest. He finally concluded that this was the most angry baby that he had ever seen. On the ride home she cried until she finally exhausted herself and us too.

Our seven year old announced in Sunday School the next Sunday that, "Mother baptized our baby and it didn't change her one little bit."

The baby was like her brother in looks (you could hardly tell their baby pictures apart). She woke up smiling and smiled all the time as long as she wasn't inconvenienced. She was a lot of fun most of the time.

As Melany grew, we also called her Missy and later Mimi. She was a fun loving delightful child and brought much love and entertainment into our family, church and the lives of our friends.

She said "MaMa" and "DaDa" at nine months old. When she was ten months old, as I rocked her and sang the lullaby, "Somewhere Over the Rainbow," she would repeat after me "birds fly" every time I said it. It was unbelievable.

She called Ric "Auga," but we didn't know why, perhaps she was trying to say "brother." By eleven months she could say "Hey there, Auga."

One day in the pediatricians office as Dr. Bennett walked in she said "Hey there, Auga." He was so astonished because he thought that she was saying "Hey there, Doctor." He called his staff in to hear her and she repeated it several times. She had become quite a little entertainer, a role that she enjoyed for years to come.

However, I did not have the heart to tell them she was not trying to say, "Hey there, Doctor." Dr. Bennett said she was the youngest child he had ever had to make a sentence. Also, he had never had one that young recognize and say doctor.

As her vocabulary increased so did her craftiness. By age two she could say anything. One of her favorite sentences was "Auga did it" This was always her reply when I would ask who had been playing in the flower pot in the living room, or splashing in the goldfish bowl. Children learn early without being taught how to put the blame on others. We moved the goldfish bowl higher after she took them out to see if they could walk.

All her life Missy loved water and enjoyed watching fish.

Missy, Ric and I were at the doctor's office one day with my mother-in-law. It was a small complex built in a semi-circle with a fish pond in the center. Ric took Melany out to watch the fish. I was watching closely from inside as he held her hand tightly. Suddenly she broke away from his grip and jumped in. Ric jumped in and got her out. Ric was nine and the water was chest deep on him so it was well over her head.

Of course I went outside right away. I was asking Ric why he turned her hand loose and she broke my grip on her little hand and jumped in again. I had on a dress, hose and high heeled shoes but I jumped in to get her. We were all soaking wet. I emerged with my cotton dress stuck to my body and a small goldfish caught in my high-heeled shoe. Melany was squealing with glee and thought this was lots of fun.

Ric asked if we had to go back in the waiting room because people were standing at the large window laughing at us. This was the first of many embarrassing instances for us and especially for him.

Melany was always interested in getting things moving forward, so she could continue to "get into the stuff" that she wanted to do. When our children were small every time they fell and bumped their head, we would ask them the following questions to be sure that they were alright.

1. "What does the dog say?"
   "Bow-wow"
2. "What does the cat say?"
   "Meow"
3. "What does the cow say?"
   "Moo"

When Melany fell, she would immediately say, "Bow-wow, Meow, Moo!"

When Ric was nine he played football for our recreation department. One evening when Melany was two she stood by the gate watching the young football players run onto the field and decided to join them. She broke from my grasp and ran behind them with her little ruffled undies just waddling over her short little legs.

People laughed and cheered as I dragged her off the field screaming. Her brother again recanted that this added to his numerous times of embarrassment.

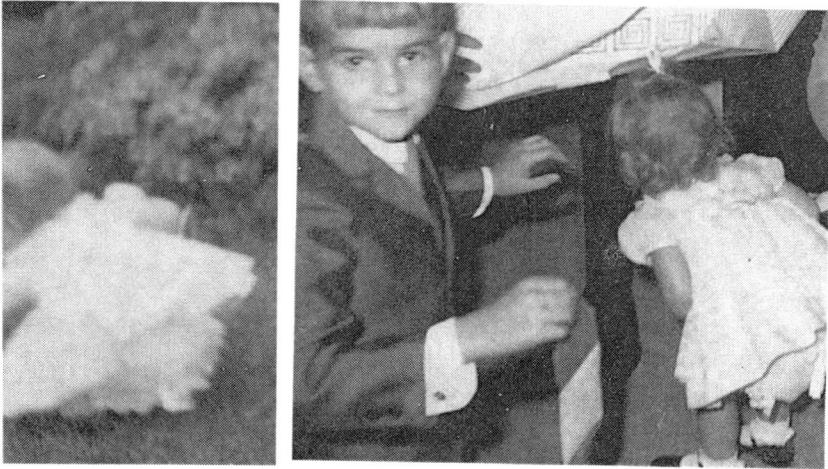

James had to work most Sundays so Ric had to "help" me corral Melany and get us all to Sunday School and church. One Sunday morning I was in the bathroom trying to finish my makeup. Missy was watching me and jumping up and down on the closed commode seat telling me to hurry because she loved to go to Sunday School.

Her foot came down and wedged between the tank on the back of the commode and the brace that holds the seat on. She did not like to be held or restricted so she began screaming loudly.

Ric ran in to help. She had on little black patent leather "Mary Jane" type shoes with a strap and a buckle. The buckle was wedged so we couldn't get her shoe off to release her. Ric tried to hold her while I got under the tank (in very close quarters). I was finally able to unscrew the seat and release the hysterical child.

The entire scenario took about thirty minutes. Ric said, "We're going to be late for Sunday School and I had a special part this morning. I'm tired, can we just stay at home?"

I told him to just explain to his teachers what had happened. He said, "I'll never tell this because they probably wouldn't believe it anyway."

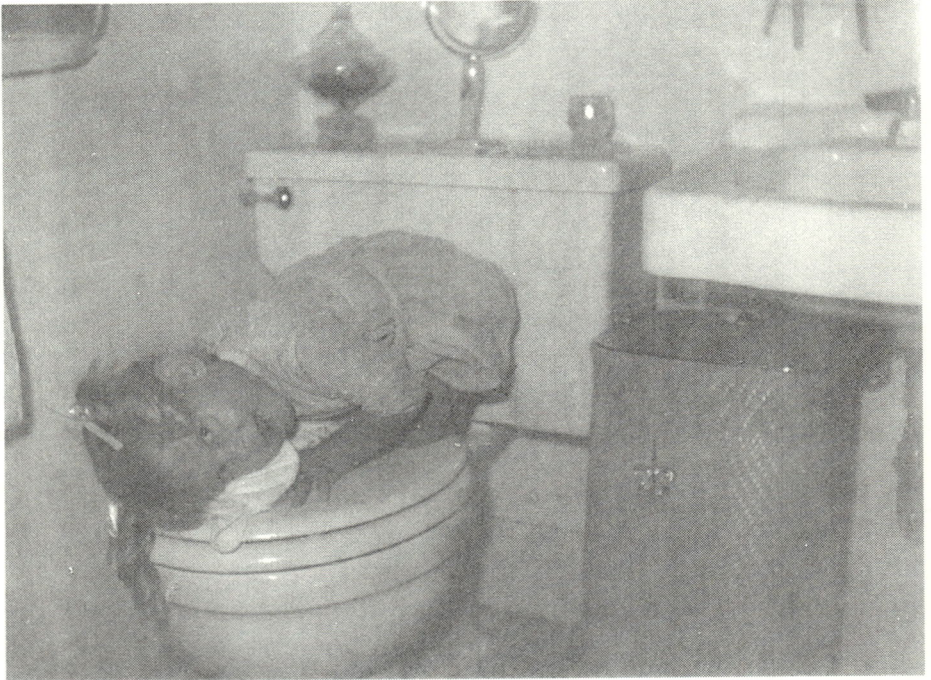

* * * * * *

I have always done the shopping for the family's clothes but one Saturday I was busy cleaning up for company. James volunteered to take Ric and Melany to buy Ric some hunting boots and then for ice cream.

They came home looking very bedraggled and a little sheepish with Ric's new hunting boots in a bag. Missy had on the brightest pair of red boots that I had ever seen. It seemed that while Ric and his dad were engrossed in choosing Ric's boots, Melany wandered over to where the little girl's boots were. When they found her (who knows how long since they had thought about her) she had a pile of boots on the floor and the red boots on her feet. It was one of those cash and carry discount shoe stores, which had both shoes connected with a plastic tape. Missy had found her a pair and put them on still connected with the plastic holder.

They tried to get them off of her feet but she screamed to the top of her lungs. Since dad was not accustomed to dealing with her antics, he tried to get her to let the sales lady check her feet to see if she had on the correct size. Perhaps fearing that if they got the boots off of her feet she would not get to keep them, she howled even louder.

Her dad who was about ten times her size did not want the embarrassment of "trying" to get them off. The manager who apparently was anxious to get this screaming child out of his store suggested that they take her shoes, leave the boots on her feet and pay for them. He said that if her mother found they did not fit he would gladly exchange them. So dad picked her up and the cashier "scanned" her feet. Ric said that everyone including the manager and the cashier was laughing, except him and his dad. They just wanted to get out of the store and come home.

They all seemed happy but mother was not. I informed the one hundred eighty pound man that he should have held her firmly and removed the boots. Then if he wanted to buy them that would have been fine.

The sheepish looking father informed me that he had tried that with the assistance of the sales-lady and the two hundred pound manager and they couldn't do it.

Then I said, "Well you should have spanked her." The ten year old said that he didn't think there were enough people in the entire store to do that. I figured that I should just drop it because they had all had a very traumatizing event except the happy three year old who wore her new boots to bed.

I was quite surprised to find that she had fitted the correct size. The next morning I informed her very emphatically that what she had done in the shoe store was what people called a temper tantrum. I said if she ever did something like this again, she would get nothing except a spanking and not the thing that she wanted.

For years later you could ask her "What does crying or pouting get you in your house?" She would always reply, "Absolutely nothing." However, she did try it from time to time.

As most youngsters do, Ric enjoyed having company spend almost every Friday night. Occasionally I would ask Ric to watch Missy for a very short time. I had done this on a particular Saturday morning while I finished cooking their breakfast. I told him and his friend to please take her into the back yard and I would bring them in to eat as soon as I was finished.

It was quite windy so I went to get Missy a jacket to hand out of the back door. The boys were playing basketball. When suddenly I heard them yelling, "Stop, stop don't run!" I bolted out the door still in my night clothes.

We had a ranch-style house with a long roof. Melany had climbed up the wrought iron supports on the carport. She was gleefully running back and forth on the roof. I was afraid that she was going to slip off. So, I climbed up the wrought iron columns and started running down the top of our very long roof. I had on a long pink robe with large billowing sleeves which the high winds caught. According to the neighbors who rushed from their yards and out of their houses to watch as traffic stopped, it looked like I was flying with a pink parachute hooked behind me. They were unable to see the little three year old who was enjoying the game as she raced over the point of the roof to the back of the house. An inquiring motorist asked if I was drunk? Our neighbor answered no, but if he had a child like that one he would be.

I finally caught her and got her down. We had only lived in the neighborhood for a couple of years. After that incident some of the neighbors viewed us as strange and referred to me as the lady who danced on the roof.

Ric's friend, Jay, who was an only child reminded him that the last time he had stayed over, Melany was watching as they were playing with the electronic football game. She had grabbed the small magnetic football, and quickly swallowed it. When I called the doctor he said, "Just don't let her get near a large magnet." Ric's friend told his mother to please never get him a sister like that. Now, he said that he really didn't want one.

Very early in Melany's life James and I felt that God had given us a special, unique child, and a special ministry in raising her. We claimed the Scripture, II Corinthians 4:1, *"Therefore, seeing we have this ministry, as we have received mercy, we faint not."* Many times we felt like fainting from embarrassment or fatigue but we didn't.

Many of the humorous and funny things that I have shared are not just to be entertaining but hopefully to be encouraging to other parents with strong-willed children. Don't give up on love, structure (as best as you can) and discipline. Be as consistent as you can, as God's word teaches us to be. However, do seek to develop a sense of humor and laughter for you will surely need it. Do not be embarrassed by what you cannot control or feel guilty by the remarks of others. Above all, try to enjoy this unique child with the feisty personality that God has given to you. These children usually have strong leadership qualities. Stay on your knees seeking God's guidance (usually praying with one eye open and watching). Always remember Jesus' words, *"My grace is sufficient for thee."* II Corinthians 12:9.

That same afternoon after the roof incident I was letting Melany help me change the water in the goldfish bowl. She asked why fish couldn't walk. We looked at the fish and talked about how God had made them to move by swimming and not walking.

I placed the four fish in a glass pyrex dish and took the bowl into the bathroom to flush the dirty water. I washed the bowl out and started back to the kitchen when I heard an excited voice saying, "Come quick Momma, the fish can't walk but they sure can fly." She had taken the fish out of the dish and placed them on the counter top. She said that they had jumped around and then they "flew" to the floor. Two of the fish survived, but they always seemed awfully nervous when Melany came around.

As parents we had determined that we would never compare our children to each other. We always encouraged them to be individuals, and to develop their own personalities.

It seemed that Missy was always into something. Between the ages of three and five anytime I asked the redundant question, "WHY did you do this?" or "What are you doing?" She would say, "I just like to prittle," or she would simply reply, "Just prittling." We were never sure what prittling was but she did an awful lot of it and it usually involved much activity, most of it not approved.

Later around the age of five she changed her answer from "prittling" to "prattling." That seemed to be a more advanced form of fun and irritation.

Melany took a nap every day after lunch. She usually slept for two full hours because she was so tired from being a human dynamo since six or seven a.m. I usually would sleep also because I was exhausted from trying to keep up with the dynamo. I would set the clock to wake up before she did because no one wanted to be asleep when she was awake and in charge of the house. One day I forgot to set the clock and I awoke and heard her playing in the hall. She often talked to herself and also to imaginary playmates. I listened and smiled as she said in a very coaxing voice, "Come on kitty, kitty, come on."

I wasn't concerned because I knew that our cat and dog were in the backyard. I had apparently slept through Missy filling up the tub with water in the front bathroom. All of a sudden I heard a splash, then the loudest commotion and noises I've ever heard.

As I stepped into the hall a slightly wet white cat ran by screeching, followed by a very wet brown dog, barking furiously. They ran through the living room, over furniture, knocking down lamps until the cat finally scampered up the draperies that covered the large sliding glass doors.

Missy stood in the middle of the living room. She loved a commotion and said very calmly, "Cats really don't like to take a bath, especially if a dog is in the tub with them."

Melany loved going to Sunday School and extended nursery at church. She had a whole new group to boss. However, she got along surprisingly well with other children and enjoyed playing and new excitement.

One Sunday morning her brother's ten-year Old choir sang and had a drama. We thought at three she would enjoy this because she loved music and certainly drama. We sat in the front of the church so she could see everything. After the drama Ric and a friend came and sat with us. Melany stayed at the end of the pew so that she could see the preacher, whom she loved very much. He and his wife had been in our home often.

Immediately after the prayer we sensed laughter behind us. Melany had taken her little "spare" pair of ruffled undies out of her little pocketbook and had put them on her head like a bonnet. As I reached for the panties, she screeched, "Stop it!" I stood up (of course her dad was at work) and as I picked her up she grabbed onto the back of the pew in front of us with a very strong grip. As soon as I would remove one hand she would grab with the other. As laughter around us erupted I finally got out into the aisle.

As I carried her out kicking she yelled, "Help Peecher Badly, Help, Peecher Badly." I don't think that Preacher Bradley was amused, however they said he did laugh.

On Wednesday Night we always ate dinner at the church. Ric had Royal Ambassadors, James and I had a class, and Missy went to the nursery. We had a new educational director who was now in charge of our activities. He announced that he was making some changes in our usual way of leaving the dinner tables and taking our children to the nursery and their mission activities. He wanted everyone to remain seated until he made the announcements.

As he started speaking Melany had finished eating and was ready to go to the nursery. Her dad whispered to her that she had to wait and she asked why? He told her that Mr. Hatfield had asked us to wait until he finished talking. She looked up at Mr. Hatfield and announced loudly (she never spoke softly), "That bald-headed man is not my peecher, and he can't tell me what to do."

She jumped out of her highchair, turned it over and ran down the hall to the nursery. I followed and took her into the restroom and swatted her backside after giving her a good talking to about her rudeness. I took her back to the dining hall and waited outside the closed door.

While we were waiting to go back in the three year-old said to me, "Don't that make you feel big? Big ole you, picking on little ole me?" This was some of her prittle. I told her that it did not make me feel big. I explained simply but firmly that God gave her parents to help her to learn to be obedient and to be kind to other people. We had this conversation several times. She held her ground, and I held mine. She told Mr. Hatfield that she was sorry and they became great friends! He said that he had never encountered such a spunky, joyful child.

Melany was very entertaining at church as well as at home. I learned early in her life that she enjoyed activity and being involved with what others were doing. When I had something that I needed to do I made sure that she had something to keep her busy, otherwise she would give me more help than I needed.

One warm sunny day the beautiful colored leaves were falling and the ground was covered with acorns. I was painting a small storage cabinet, and she was painting boards and a box full of acorns with her tray of colored washable paints. It takes a three year old a long time to paint a box of acorns.

I went into the kitchen to answer the phone. We didn't have the luxury of cordless phones then. I watched her out the kitchen window while I was having a brief conversation. She was sitting in the same place, dipping her paint brush, and painting intently. What I could not see until I got to the back door was that she was painting our neighbor's long haired Persian cat.

She was holding the cat tightly by the tail and had streaked his back with orange and yellow paint. I grabbed an old towel and briskly rubbed his back which made his long hair bristle up in a weird way. The frightened cat broke away, jumped our back fence and ran home.

I quickly called our vet, told him what had happened and asked if the child's washable paint would harm the cat. He laughed (everyone laughed except us and the owner of the cat) and said that the cat should be bathed immediately.

I knew for sure I was not going to try to bathe a large cat that had just been held and painted by a three year old. I called my neighbor and amid her hysterical screams at seeing her cat, I offered to pay for her to take her traumatized cat to the vet to be checked and bathed. She said some very unkind things to me and concluded by asking, "What kind of a child do you have that would paint a cat?"

I was thinking the same thing and meekly responded, "One that stays in her own yard." We never saw that cat again. He was either too scared of Missy or too ashamed to be seen in public.

At the age of four the children in our church must go into the sanctuary, or "big church" as the little ones called it and Melany was very anxious to go. We definitely felt that she was better off in the extended session where she could play and talk and we knew that the rest of the congregation was, too.

The entire family dreaded the day that Missy had to go to big church. We thought about doing a trial run and see how she would do. We all remembered that last fiasco. So we decided to wait until we had to take her and she did surprisingly well. She enjoyed the singing and sang quite loudly. She observed everything around her and behaved fine.

After her first Sunday morning experience, her grandmother asked her what she liked most about the service. She quickly replied, "The bald-headed angels." Since we had all been in the same service and none of us had seen any angels, bald or with hair, we started questioning her. Finally she said, "They sat in front of us. Then they walked by us with pans and took our money. They went out the door and flew it to God." Her eleven year old brother said, "Wow, this gets better all the time. Baldheaded angels stealing our money and flying it to God. That sounds more like Robin Hood."

Missy was getting very perturbed with us. It was for sure that she had seen something that had made an impression on her. She could remember it well and couldn't understand why we couldn't. Then I remembered when the deacons were taking up the offering she had asked, "What are they doing?" I had whispered, "They are the deacons (the church helpers) and they are taking the money for Jesus." Missy had a vivid imagination so I'm sure that she filled in the rest which made perfect sense to her.

We have always felt the children behaved better when they sat near the front of the church. Where they could see the choir and the preacher. It seemed to work well for our children and our friends did the same with theirs. We sat on the side of the church near the side door so that if we had to leave (and we often did) we would be less distracting.

We sat on the first pew behind the deacons. Melany waved at all of them as they entered the side door and they would smile at her, especially the ones that knew her. We were horrified to learn from one of our deacon friends several weeks later that during prayers Missy had poked one of them with a pencil, put a paper clip down two of their shirt collars, and poked her finger in several ears. They had all compared their experiences our friend had said laughingly. After that I always prayed with one eye open and I believe some of the deacons did too.

We had renovated our sanctuary and added a large crescent

shaped altar rail. Our pastor would invite people to come to the altar during prayer call. We always went forward because we certainly needed prayer and wanted to pray for others. We had explained to Missy why we went there to pray. She had already developed a growing little prayer life and loved to pray.

We were at the altar on our knees praying when I realized that Missy was no longer beside me. I looked to either side then up to the pulpit. Preacher Bradley was standing in the center, with Missy right beside him, smiling brightly. He had a portable mike, and as he walked back and forth she walked with him. I motioned for her to come to me but she shook her head covered with long golden curls, smiled and looked the other way.
By this time others had become aware that there was a child walking with the preacher. Preacher Bradley signaled for me to just stay where I was. As the prayers ended he grasped her hand and walked toward me, picked her up and handed her over the rail.

Missy immediately screeched to the top of her lungs. As I exited the side door carrying her she was squealing, "I just want to help Peecher Badly, I just want to help!" It's hard to spank a child that just wants to help the preacher! When we got out into the side vestibule I sat her down and explained that the preacher did not need help with the prayer call and that she had been quite disruptive. I told her that I was not happy one little bit, nor were the people who were trying to talk to God.

I also informed her (I did a lot of informing), that we were going back into the church for the remaining part of the service and that she was to sit down and be quiet or she would get a spanking. She assured me that she would be good and asked, "Momma, does God still love me?" I told her that God had always loved her and that he always would. I further explained (to a four year old) that God was not happy when we misbehaved, but that God and her mother and daddy would always love her.

We waited at the door until the soloist finished singing and the preacher stood up to preach. As we walked in Missy smiled angelically. She looked toward the preacher, waved with her free hand and said very loudly, "Hi, peecher, God still loves me."

The preacher smiled and nodded his head. I wanted to leave again and go home but I humbly went back to our pew and sat down. Missy was very good for the rest of that service. On the ride home Ric asked why didn't we just stay at home until she was older. We really were tempted but we had promised to raise this child in the church. We believed Proverbs 22:6, "*Train up a child in the way he should go; and when he is old, he will not depart from it.*"

The next Sunday at altar call we went back with a stern warning about misbehaving. We knelt on the side of the large group away from the preacher and near the door. Our associate pastor's wife, Joan, and I had their four year old Rusty, and my Missy corralled between us. The prayers that day were longer than usual and we realized at the same time that both children were nowhere to be seen. We motioned to each other that we had not heard the side door open so apparently they were still in this great throng of people. Then we panicked because the doors at the back of our sanctuary open on to our busiest downtown street.

Joan and I stood up and backed against the side wall. We searched for two little heads trying to be as inconspicuous as possible. We noticed that there seemed to be a slight commotion on the side of the church where we were standing. The people in each pew were looking down and smiling.

Joan and I immediately went up the side aisle disrupting prayers I'm sure. We were standing in the open space at the back of the pews when two little figures wiggled out side by side from under the last pew. They had crawled on their stomachs through the feet and under the pews to what they thought was going to be freedom.

Joan and I agreed on how we disciplined our children. We always calmly explained to our children why they were being punished, punished them, then assured them of our love. That day we forgot our own rules. With the rush of fear that only a parent can experience when a child is missing, combined with great embarrassment; we snatched them out the back door. When outside, we immediately paddled the two little chums in mischief.

We returned to the last pew in the church and sat there holding two unhappy young escapees. Joan's husband, Don was standing on the pulpit with Dr. Bradley and was observing the entire episode. He told us later we were scowling, looking like two mean drill sergeants which even scared him.

Later Joan and I discussed the situation involving our energetic children. We claimed II Chronicles 20:12, *"Neither know we what to do. But our eyes are upon Thee."*

The next week Joan and I went to the pastor and asked if they could please start a children's church at least through the third grade. He laughed and was glad to oblige. I also told our preacher that I would just pray in my pew and not be going back to the altar call until we had children's church. He agreed that was a good idea.

We had a few more rough spots while they were getting children's church organized and securing workers. Amazingly it only took a month to get it together.

During that month our pastor had several spot appeals on our local TV station inviting people to our church. One Saturday evening as we were doing our regular hair rolling (to make long beautiful curls instead of frizzy hair) the TV message came on.

It showed our church in the background with a close up of our pastor. Dr. Bradley smiled and said, "This is Lawrence Bradley inviting you to attend (with the emphasis he made he pronounced it a-ten) church services with us this Sunday." As he continued Missy jumped up and cried, "Oh no, not ten church services tomorrow. I can't stand that. I can't hardly make it through one." I assured her that Dr. Bradley would not have her to sit through ten services.

"I am born happy every morning!"
<u>*(Apples of Gold*</u>)

"God trusts us with these frail little beings, tender and impressionable, perhaps so that we will more fully recognize our need for Him in this venture."

"By using kind words and a pleasant tone of voice in the face of frustration and delay,   We speak volumes to our children about choosing patience."
<u>*(Parenting the Way God Parents)*</u>

CHAPTER II
PRATTLE

"Ye rejoice with Joy unspeakable and full of glory." I Peter 1:8b

"Then were there brought unto Him little children that He should put His hands on them, and pray; And the disciples rebuked them. But Jesus said, "Suffer little children and forbid them not to come unto me; for of such is the Kingdom of Heaven." Matthew 19:13-14.

Melany continued to be her usual joyful self at home and church. The night her brother's friend Chris was baptized was special to all of us. We had explained baptism to her. Missy only had to be reprimanded once during the worship service because she was hanging her black patent leather shoes on her ears and sitting up like a little puppy dog begging.

During the solemn baptismal service Melany sat very still and was very observant. Dr. Bradley made comments to Chris concerning what baptism meant to his life and immersed him in the the water and brought him back up. Overcome with emotional glee Missy called out, "Dunk him again 'peecher', dunk him again!"

Our pastor told us after Missy was going to children's church that he really missed her. I'm sure that he did! He said that he enjoyed her spontaneity and the fact that she was always joyful. Also he knew she loved him, because she told him just about every time he saw her.

Of course she continued to go to worship on Sunday nights. Usually she was tired after a full day of activity (with a short nap) and went to sleep right after the singing.

As Missy neared the age of five she developed some very pleasing qualities. She deeply loved and expressed love to family members and friends. She had many little friends and shared her toys and things willingly. She would always tell the truth even when she knew she would be punished.

As a family we read the Bible and prayed every evening. Missy had mimicked me by telling people "I'll be praying for you," then she would remember to call their names in prayer. She prayed for everyone, a wonderful habit that she had as long as she lived, even her last day on this earth. Every night she would pray for our family members, friends, doctors, our pastor and staff (she knew them all), neighbors and the trash men. She always closed her prayer by saying, "And God bless me." He always did and continued to do so as long as she lived.

We had enjoyed wonderful neighbors for several years. The Hudelson's-Jerry, Bonnie and their two little girls, Debbie and Dianne. They enjoyed many of Melany's escapades before they moved to Washington State. The summer before Melany was five we had new neighbors move in next door to us. They were a lovely family and we all became very close especially Missy and Dianne who was four also. They both had the same type personality and determination and got along very well. James said they had an animal instinct of how far they could push each other. They immediately became cohorts in mischief. The oldest child was a boy named Michael who was the same age as Ric. They were great buddies, and shared the same interests. Their middle child nine year old Donna, was a good helper to Bernadine and me as we tried to keep up with Missy and Dianne.

We had a small very shallow creek (or stream) at the back of our yards. Ric and his friends had played in the stream for years and later Melany and her friends did too. We had installed a high fence between the play area in the back yard and the creek. We had a walk through gate that stayed locked unless we were in the back yard. Even though we watched them carefully and constantly we certainly wanted all the protection that we could provide.

When Melany and Dianne were playing in the creek then Bernadine or I stayed in our back yards. We both got a lot of yard work done and good suntans. The stream was only knee deep on them, but we took no chances with those two.

Bernadine had yard duty one day while Missy and Dianne were playing in the creek and she heard the girls squealing (they did that a lot) and laughing. All of a sudden Missy's large white cat streaked past hissing and squawking as displeased cats do. Upon investigating she found that the girls had "baptized" the poor cat two times before he got away.

That night at the supper table her daddy asked Missy, "Baby, how in the world did two little girls like you and Dianne baptize that large cat?" She laid her knife and fork down and raised her right hand and solemnly said, "In the name of the Father, the Son and the Holy Spirit."

We told her that cats, even large ones like Snowball, did not like water. Then we talked to her about being kind to animals and never mistreating them. Also, that she was never to baptize any more animals. She said, "But Daddy, don't you want them to go to Heaven?" James assured her that we did and that God would surely take care of them.

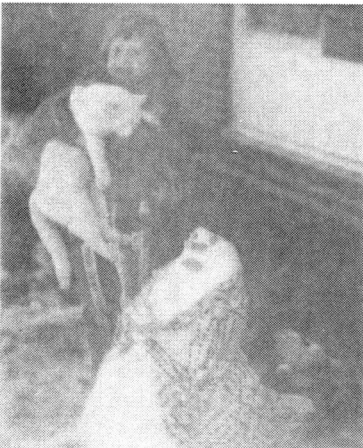

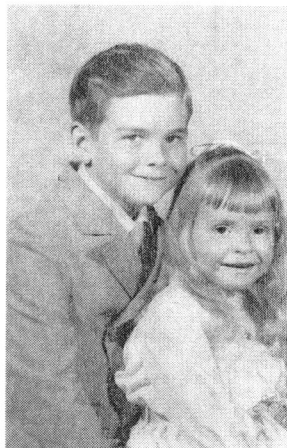

Melany with large white cat (left) and Ric and Melany.

Missy's self-coined word "prittle" changed to "prattle" Sometime around her fifth birthday. Then she would say, "Oh, I'm just prattling." or "I just like to prattle." Prattling was definitely an advanced form of prittling and involved a lot more activity which continued well into her school life.

As soon as Melany was five in January she was ready to go to kindergarten. Explaining to her that she could not go until September was not what she wanted to hear. She and Dianne had been enrolled in a three-day a week play school since September which they enjoyed with lots of activities but they wanted to go to "real school."

The summer before kindergarten was very busy for Missy. She could already read quite well and told me one day she knew the "Rotor-Rooter's" phone number. I replied that was nice.

I had to go to the doctor and was leaving Missy with our maid. I forgot my check book so I came back in about five minutes. As soon as I came in the door Missy was encouraging me to hurry up and leave so I wouldn't be late. I became a little suspicious so I purposefully lingered.

The phone rang and I answered it in the kitchen. As soon as I said, "Hello, Mr. Brown," Missy dashed out the back door. Mr. Brown was the owner of our local "Rotor-Rooter" Company. We had to use him often for several of our rental houses and Melany would go with me while they were doing their service. She loved to watch the large rotor open up the sewer lines.

We had pine trees in the front of our house and had to have our sewer lines reamed out a couple of times a year. I would make Missy stay in the house and watch out her front bedroom window and she thoroughly enjoyed this adventure. Mr. Brown would always play with her through the window and she knew him well.

Mr. Brown said a lot of working mothers would have their children call during the day for their services and they tried to check on these calls. His secretary had become a little suspicious when she knew that the caller was a very young one and even more so when she gave very good directions to the house (as she had heard me do many times on the phone). Then she added, "Don't come to the door, just turn on your rotor and start rooting."

As I apologized for her behavior, (as I often did) Mr. Brown asked, "Mrs. Wiggins was it that little girl that poked all the miniature pool balls down your commode that time? If you remember, it was packed so tight that we had to remove the bowl to get them out." Indeed I did remember it! I answered that she was the same one and he said, "She surely is a live wire, isn't she?" Indeed she was!

As I said earlier, Melany and Dianne had the same type personalities and the same determination to have things go as they wanted. Everyone was surprised that they got along so well and they worked out their disagreements. Sometimes they slugged them out but both had a real sense of fairness and very tender little hearts.

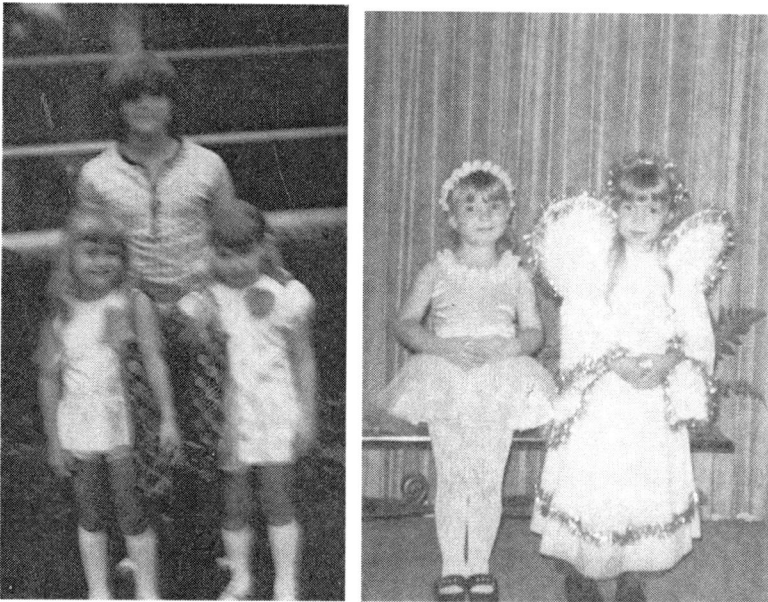

Ric with Melany and Dianne Skains (left);
Dianne (ballet) and Melany (angel) at Halloween (right)

One summer day the dog catcher came into our neighborhood looking for a stray dog someone had reported as being sick. They parked their truck in the street between our houses. It was filled with approximately ten to fifteen dogs. The truck had heavy wire screen on both sides and a latch on the back door. The driver and helper were walking through the neighbors' yards searching for the stray dog.

Of course Missy and Dianne went to investigate the situation. Their older brothers, Ric and Mike loved to get the girls upset and they told them the men were taking the dogs to doggie prison and most of them would be put to sleep. There was probably some truth there, but five year-olds didn't need to hear that especially highly emotional, tender hearted ones.

The girls screamed loudly and started hitting the boys who were laughing hysterically. Then together they calmly walked to the back of the truck and lifted the latch lock. As they opened the cage door, about ten to fifteen happy dogs leaped out and bounded away in every direction.

Bernadine and I turned and walked into our houses we didn't want to see the dog catcher, the girls came in very proud of what they had done. Their brothers followed and Mike said, "Do you think they are going to be juvenile delinquents?"

Bernadine and I looked at each other in horror!

That night Missy and Ric reported the incident to their dad, including Mike's question. He said that he certainly hoped not. After the children were in bed James and I had our nightly talk.

We asked the Lord again as we had so many times to help us guide this little energetic, caring being in the way that He would have her to go. James and I also told the Lord that He knew that we often got frustrated and sometimes scared about her future because of her determination.

James found these two verses of Scripture and shared them with me.

"*Concerning the work of my hands, command Ye me.*" Isaiah 45:11.

"*When thou goest, thy way shall be opened up before thee step by step."* Proverbs 4:12 (Free translation).

Then we knew that the Lord would direct us as we sought him. We just had to trust Him, step by step.

Our family always went to the beach for a week every summer and had great fun. One year our friends Bobbie and Frank McKnight and their two sons went with us. Missy decided that she was ready to learn to swim. With the same determination that she exhibited toward everything she persevered until she learned.

As we were driving home James mentioned that it was about time for his cousin and his family to visit us. They usually came every summer for a few days either on the way to the mountains in North Georgia, or on their return home. However, they never let us know in advance.

I made the remark that with all the dirty clothes and all of the sand on us I really hoped that they didn't come today. I forgot about the conservation as we came home and started unloading all the luggage and dirty clothes and towels (we didn't have a washing machine and dryer at the beach).

I saw a new car I did not recognize drive up in front of our house. James, Ric and Missy were standing by the car as I walked to the front door. Missy yelled loudly, "Momma, it's those people that you said you hoped didn't come." We apologized and tried to explain what I meant but I am not sure they ever really believed us. Missy always spoke her mind.

Missy continued "prattling" through the summer just waiting for kindergarten to start. She and Dianne were so excited. Bernadine and I took them shopping and bought identical school supplies. They had several fights before they agreed on each item.

Finally the time came for kindergarten. Bernadine and I told them we would take them the first day and then they could ride the big yellow bus with Ric, Mike and Donna. They both insisted that they wanted to ride the bus the very first day and could find their teachers without our help or the help of their siblings. Their siblings didn't want anyone to know that they were kin to them, so that was fine.

We had requested that they be placed in separate classes, because we didn't feel it was fair for one teacher to have to "put up" with those two. For identification Dianne had been sent a bird made out of construction paper and Melany had a fish. They had their names and their teachers' names printed on them. They said they would just go to the gym and look for the fish and the birds.

As soon as Bernadine and I put our small babies on the large yellow bus we drove to the school. We watched the big bus arrive and Missy and Dianne jump off of the bottom step side by side. They gleefully ran into the gym and by the time Bernadine and I arrived they had found the fish and the birds and were eager to go to their classes.

Missy's energy level seemed to increase after she started to kindergarten. After being confined from nine to twelve, she would come home, eat lunch, take a nap and wake up wide open and was busy prattling until bedtime. One afternoon when I had endured enough prattling I said to her, "Missy, Mrs. McKnight says that you are very cooperative in her class. Why do you misbehave so badly at home? I know you don't act like this in school."

Without a pause she replied, "Well, I thought about that and I decided that I couldn't be good all the time. I figured that you had rather me be bad at home and good away from home, instead of being good at home and bad away from home." I decided that if I had to make a choice that would be it.

Missy learned a lot of things that year in kindergarten. She already knew her ABCs and could count to one hundred by fives and tens. She learned very important stuff such as how to sit still for a little while, how to cooperate, and how to get along with others (most of the time). The thing that made her most proud was she learned to "spit." It took a long time for us to help her unlearn that. I think that she finally just got tired of doing it.

Melany liked to be in control of things and she really was a great organizer. One day her little friend and neighbor, Mary who had been her friend since they were two and three, came into the kitchen crying. She said that Melany had spanked her because she wouldn't do what Missy wanted. I explained to her that she did not have to do what Melany told her. Mary was taller and heavier than Missy and I told her, "Don't let her hit you, just sit on her and call me." I was usually within hearing distance.

Mary continued, "When we are at my house Melany tells me that I have to do what her wants because her is company. When we are here her says that I have to do what her says because it's her house."

Mary couldn't figure out all of this. She knew one thing for sure, they always did what Missy wanted, and she never got her way. Melany enjoyed getting her own way and usually did except with Dianne.

Melany had an uncanny sense of fairness and would promptly belt anyone regardless of their size who cheated. We just had to help her begin the learning process of her being fair. Soon she was a lot better at it, and would take turns giving Mary her way. Mary also got a little more assertive but of course that brought more disharmony.

During her kindergarten year Melany also learned about jealousy. Being seven years apart in age our children both had plenty of our undivided attention in their early years. They had never really been jealous of each other. Of course as they got older they had the normal sibling rivalry but not jealousy. Also, neither one seem to have a jealous nature.

Around Christmas time Missy met the green-eyed monster also known as the Big J. Dianne had stayed home from kindergarten to go to a doctor's appointment. When Missy came in from school and had finished her nap I had to tell her the earth-shattering news. Dianne had gotten her ears pierced and

Nancy Wiggins

had pretty little gold posts in her ears. She had run over to show them to me and said that she would come back when Melany got up from her nap. I knew that I had to prepare Melany for this visit.

When I gave Missy the news she just fell out in the floor sobbing. "Why can't I, why can't I get my ears pierced?" she repeated. I sat down with her and gently explained (for what seemed like the fiftieth time) why we didn't let her get her ears pierced yet.

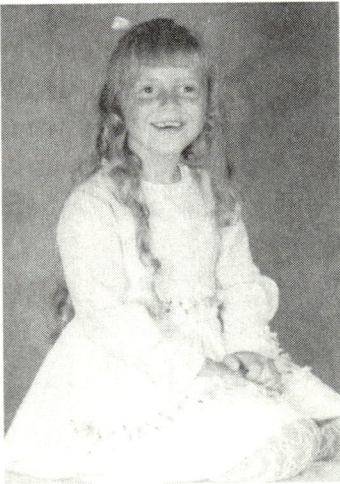

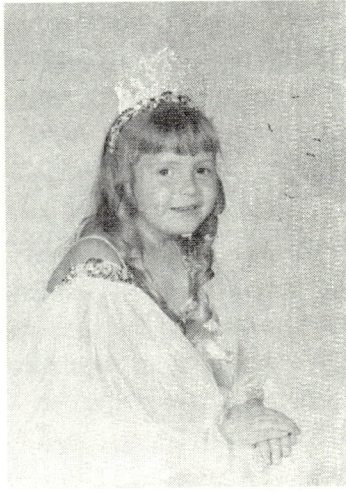

**Melany at age 5 (top left), Melany in ballet garb (top right)
Melany dressed for tap (below)**

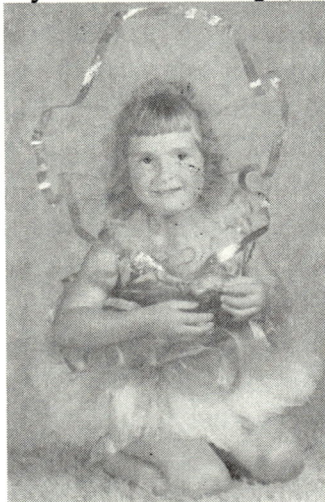

We wanted our children to look forward to their teenage years, and enjoy some special things then. For our son we made him wait until he was thirteen to have certain name brand shoes and jeans that everyone had, and to have a special expensive ball glove that he wanted. He really enjoyed and appreciated these things when he got them.

For Missy it was that she could wear hose and have her ears pierced when she was thirteen. She would also get name brands if she desired.

We explained to them that there's not a lot of things a young teenager can look forward to while they wait for the magical age of sixteen, when they get their drivers license and more freedom. The younger ones can usually have a later bedtime and be allowed to make a few more choices about their life.

We simply wanted them to have a few enjoyable things to look forward to. If they had already had these few pleasures when they were younger, they might feel bored and start looking for exciting experiences in drinking, drugs, smoking, etc.

We expressed to them that these were simply our ideas and rules. Other parents might allow these things, because they were not bad things, it just wasn't our choices or what we wanted for them.

Ric had never fought these ideas. Missy had wanted her ears pierced since age three so I knew that this was going to be tough for her.

I said, "Missy, I know how badly you want pierced ears and I know that you are upset that Dianne has had hers done. Now you need to think about this when you see Dianne if you are angry and pout and act mean this will hurt her feelings and you can lose a good friend." "Or you can say 'Your earrings are pretty,' because they really are and make your friend happy." I told her this was a big girl choice and she should think about it and ask God to help her do the right thing.

Missy went over to Dianne's and stayed for a little while and she returned and announced "Well I did it. I told her that her earrings were pretty."

I complimented her on doing the right thing. Then I asked, "And how did that make you feel? Didn't you feel good in your heart?"

Missy looked at me very seriously, then she said very sternly, "No, something in here," (placing her hand on her chest) "said, brurrrr." With that statement she turned her hand round and round in a twirling motion.

I have often thought about this conversation. I believe that this five year-old's explanation is the best description of jealousy that I have ever heard. Jealousy can cause a whirling sensation in our chest and mind; for some stronger than for others. If we don't work on conquering it, it can lead to stronger emotions of anger and bitterness.

Of course I did not try to explain all of that to a five year-old. She had learned about jealousy and apparently she learned to handle it in her own way because she was never a jealous, angry or bitter person. Although later in her life, she could have used her illness and disability as justification to have had a little of all three.

As I said earlier, I only wish that God had let me know that she would need all of that determination, energy, and strong will just to survive. He didn't but He just said for me to trust Him, to love her, and to teach her to love and trust Him. Missy continued to be a joyful child and a real joy in our lives.

At an early age Missy was like a little spiritual sponge. She seemed to absorb scripture verses, prayer and principals and things of the Lord. She expressed her love for God and was eager to please Him (most of the time). Once when she was being especially difficult, I said to her, "Missy when you are cooperative with your mother and mind me and behave yourself, then you please Jesus. When you misbehave and act up so badly, you please the devil. Now tell me, who do you want to please?"

She immediately answered, "Sometimes I want to please Jesus and sometimes I want to please the devil." What child-like honesty! I think we are all really like that sometimes but we will never admit it because we want to do what we want.

Although Melany behaved better in kindergarten, she was still the class clown and enjoyed fun. At the open house before Christmas we sat in our children's seats, and would stand when our names were called. When Melany's name was called the other parents laughed and clapped. They knew HER!

"I want a soul (life) so full of joy--
Life's withering storms cannot destroy."
<u>*(Apples of Gold)*</u>

"Limits that are firm make children feel more comfortable, even safer.
Limits that are weak make children feel unsafe and insecure."

"Perhaps it is when I am at the end of my parental rope that God is happiest, because He knows that my next step is to turn toward Him."
<u>*(Parenting the Way God Parents)*</u>

CHAPTER III
PAIN

"PERFECT THROUGH SUFFERING." HEBREWS 2:10

*"FOR I RECKON THAT THE SUFFERINGS OF THIS PRESENT
TIME ARE NOT WORTHY TO BE COMPARED WITH THE
GLORY WHICH SHALL BE REVEALED IN US."
ROMANS 8:18*

During kindergarten, first, and second grade Missy wanted to be involved in everything. Dianne, Mary and Missy were in music, ballet, tap, gymnastics, cheerleading and, of course, choir and GAs at church. These activities used a lot of their energy but Missy did it all. We tried to keep her busy but not over stimulated. She loved doing everything. She found time to be very creative and plenty of time for prittling and prattling.

Teachers, family and friends often said, "It never rains on her parade." But the storm clouds came, and turned into boisterous gales of winds, shattering dreams. They were like tornados, striking relentlessly with unbelievable pain, again and again for over 30 years.

In kindergarten and first grade Missy had reoccurring bladder infections. They were always treated promptly and in first grade the doctor had stretched her urethra a couple of times but that did not help.

In second and third grades she would have long occurrences of swelling in her ankles, feet and hands. At times the pain was so great that she could not even pick up her feet. She could only shuffle them along. She often had to wear her bedroom slippers because of the pain and swelling. She had great difficulty holding a pencil because of the pain in her fingers and hands.

Still she did all of her work with great determination. From first through twelfth grade she never made a grade below an A.

The doctors treated her for juvenile arthritis. She finally had to give up dancing, softball and cheerleading. She devoted a lot of her time to her piano playing, and other musical instruments despite an enormous amount of pain.

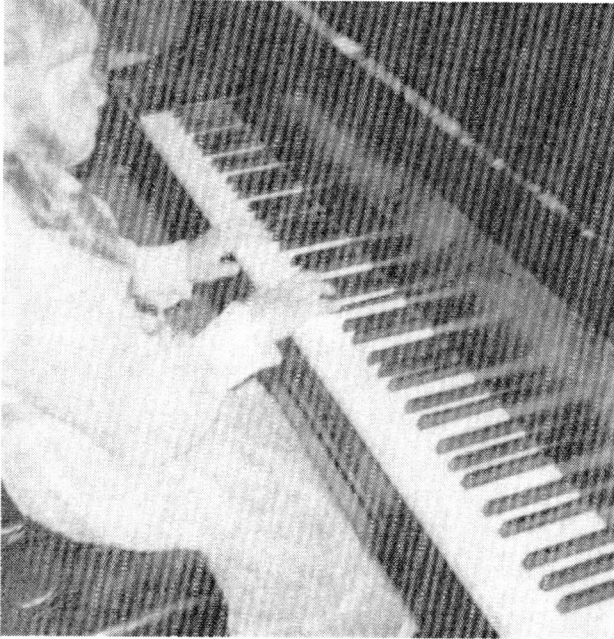

Missy remained as active as she could. She started having seizure like episodes, usually after recess or any type of exertion. They could not determine what was wrong. They did the usual tests and put her on seizure medication which didn't seem to help.

One day the father of one of her classmates came to get his daughter from school during recess. He was a pediatrician and witnessed Missy having one of her seizures. He had the teacher call for an ambulance. Even though she came to and seemed fine before the ambulance arrived he sent her to the hospital. He called her pediatrician and told him that her heart had actually stopped but it had started back.

They called me and I went immediately to the hospital. They kept her in the hospital and did many tests. They found that she had tachycardia. They also found that something in her brain would tell her heart that she was "running up hill" when she was actually sitting still.

We had now added a cardiologist, a gynecologist and a neurologist to her pediatrician and orthopedist. The doctors suggested that we limit her activities. We had already done this and it helped some with her heart problem. Her heart would still just begin racing wildly, and she would lie down, at home or at school.

Melany had begun having ulcers in her mouth, throat, urethra, her private area, and her rectum. They were very painful and she would miss days from school. She was hospitalized many times and was treated with massive doses of prednisone and other steroids.

The gynecologist started cauterizing the many ulcers. One time they counted over fifty from the size of a pin head to the size of a small eraser. The doctor's theory was the cauterization would make a small burn or blister, and that would heal the ulcerated skin, which they treated with some kind of purple liquid and with topical creams. They did this three days a week for a month.

The process was excruciatingly painful especially for an eight year old girl. I had to take her to the doctor's office every day. Missy would start crying and begging not to go. It would break my heart. I tried to explain to her that although this was painful the doctors hoped that it would help her to heal and she would not have this condition anymore.

I would often have to wait until her fifteen year old brother got home from school. He would help me get her into the car but would beg me not to take her. It hurt him so badly to know what she was experiencing. Once he went back into the house after helping me bodily put her in the car and rammed his fist through the breakfast room door.

His dad did not punish him, he simply said, "Son, I know exactly how you feel. But we cannot express our pain and anger this way."

As we drove out of the neighborhood, we would see her friends playing in their yards. Missy would start begging, "Momma, please don't make me go. I will do anything that you want me to do. I'll be good the rest of my life, if you just won't make me go."

Her request would rend my heart and I would tell her that she wasn't doing anything wrong. I wasn't punishing her but was trying to help her. All the while my heart was aching and I was wishing that I could take her back home.

Missy tried to be a brave little girl. She would go into the waiting room and then into the treatment room but they wouldn't let me go in with her. They tried to numb the area but it was still very painful. When the treatments were over she would come out crying or sniffling. I would put my arms around her and weep with her. I would tell her that I was so sorry that we had to let her go through this.

Most of the time as we were riding home she would sit close to me and respond to the comfort that I offered but occasionally she would be so hurt physically and emotionally that she would pull away from me and not want me to touch her. That really hurt me. I longed to comfort her but she refused me.

Many times in speaking engagements I have used this example in relationship to God's sovereignty. I as a finite parent allowed my child, whom I loved more than life itself, to go through great pain. Ultimately I hoped it would be for her good.

Often our all wise and infinite Heavenly Father allows us to go through great pain and difficulty. He knows that it is for our good, according to His divine purpose, if we will just commit it to Him, and trust Him. His desire is for us to come to Him in our pain for His comfort.

We make all kind of promises to God. If He will just remove our pain then we will be good. We'll serve Him, we'll change our life, we'll tithe, and on and on we go. But God doesn't remove our pain whether physical or emotional because he is not punishing us. He is trying to help us to become more like Him, and preparing us to be used for His glory.

Often we respond to God by drawing closer to Him and letting Him be the source of our comfort. But at other times we are hurt or angry and we pull away and refuse His comfort and consolation. How that must grieve our Father's heart!

God always controls the circumstances of our lives. We control our responses whether they help us grow or cause us to become bitter.

Archbishop Leighton says,

> *"Extraordinary afflictions are not always*
> *the punishment of extraordinary sins,*
> *But sometimes the trial of*
> *Extraordinary graces."*

All her life Missy had loved for me to sing two songs as she was going to sleep. I would sing, "Somewhere Over the Rainbow," and all the verses of "Jesus Loves Me." When she was real sick or in pain, then she would want me to repeat the last two stanzas:

> *"Jesus loves me, He will stay,*
> *Close beside me all the way.*
> *If I love Him when I die,*
> *He will take me home on high."*
> *"Jesus loves me, loves me still,*
> *Though I'm little, weak and ill.*
> *From His shining throne on high,*
> *Comes to watch me where I lie."*

One night she said, "Mother, tell me again what Heaven is like." We talked about what a wonderful place it was. Then she said, "If Heaven is like everyone says, why do we want to stay here? Sometimes when I hurt so bad I think about how good it would be to be with Jesus and my grand-daddies and not have any pain." Missy was only eight years old. She had thirty three more years of pain. I have often had that same thought myself.

Pain continued to be an almost daily part of her life for many years and she missed a lot of school. We spent many long and painful hours in doctors' offices every week.

I am a very patient person, and try to be understanding with others. But it disturbs me to hear people complaining about having to wait in a medical facility or a doctors' office. I remember a Medical Missionary once telling that in the bush country where he had his hospital and office that many times patients would have to walk a day's journey just to get to his facility. He told of a mother who started walking with a two year old and a small baby. The journey took her almost two days and was very difficult. On the way the baby died, the little mother dug a shallow grave with her hands and buried the little body, covering it with grass and leaves so the animals wouldn't devour it. I've never forgotten that message but often think how can I possibly complain when we must wait (usually in comfortable circumstances) for the wonderful health care that we get here in America. I shared that story with Melany, because we had a lot of long waits, often having to see several doctors in one day.

Missy's prittle and prattle did slow down a bit but her good spirits and determination continued. She was a little bit of a girl but she wasn't afraid of anything.

The doctors just did not know what was wrong with her and spent long hours trying to get a correct diagnosis. They simply had to treat the myriad symptoms as they would arise.

She was in the hospital approximately forty times by the time she was ten years old. She had four myelograms and eight spinal taps during one year. Dr. Pomeroy Nichols was an excellent, caring neurologist. He came home from his vacation a day early to do one of her myelograms himself.

The Thanksgiving that she was ten, she had been in the

hospital for three months. As our family (some from out of town), gathered in the hospital dining room for our Thanksgiving Dinner we felt that Melany was improving and hopefully would be able to go home for Christmas.

The week after Thanksgiving, the doctors let Melany go home. She couldn't wait to put up the Christmas Trees. Through the years we had put up six Christmas Trees, so that wherever Melany was, she could see a tree.

This year we only had two. Ric had already decorated the one in the small den, off of the living room. We were hoping Melany could come home to decorate the large family tree in the large den that joined her bedroom. It was placed on the upper level, so she could view it from the bed through the double doors. Her Dad and brother had the artificial tree up, and the lights and decorations were ready to place on the tree. She watched as they put on the lights, then we pushed her wheelchair up close so that she could put on her special ornaments.

Through the years we had given our children a small inexpensive, shiny gold plated ornament each year with their name and the date on it. One day we hoped that they would enjoy having these on their own trees, hopefully reminding them of many happy Christmas times.

It had become a tradition. They would put their special ornaments on, then add the other decorations. When Melany had placed three of her ornaments on, she had to go back to bed. Ric didn't want to put his on until she finished, so we decided to wait until tomorrow, hoping it would surely be a better day.

The next morning at daybreak, after a long, hard night her temperature was 104. As we drove out of the driveway taking her back to the hospital, we all had heavy hearts, because we felt she would not be back home before Christmas, if at all!

That night after they had Melany settled into the regular routine, and her fever was down, she went to sleep. I sat for a while by the decorated tree in the waiting room near her room. They had said that her dad could bring a small artificial tree the next day, but we couldn't have lights on it, because of the sensitive machines in the hospital. I promised her that when she got back home, even if it was after Christmas, that we would have a lighted Christmas Tree in all twelve rooms of our house, as well as the three bathrooms. The next year, and every one thereafter, we did. This was the first of five hospital stays through the Christmas Season. The first one was probably the most difficult.

As I sat in silence, I thought about the coming Holidays. I had many wonderful memories, and assorted thoughts.

Last year if you had asked me during this blessed season, what did I really worship at Christmas, the Truth of Christmas, or the Traditions of Christmas. I would have replied without hesitation, The Truth. For the Birth of Christ was only the beginning of a marvelous process that brought us an example of a perfect God-like life; a cruel thankless death that paid in full our debt for all of our sins. His resurrection promises us eternal life in Heaven with Him, our loved ones and friends gone before us. Through the years that has given us sustaining grace for every situation in our lives. His Holy Spirit gives us direction and comfort everyday and in all difficult circumstances.

Now I was thinking about the wonderful Traditions that we had always enjoyed with our families and friends. I realized now that for many years, my Christmas Celebration had indeed been a precious combination of Truth and Tradition.

As I contemplated the real meaning of Christmas: Joy, Peace, Hope, I sorted it out as picked up God's Word, and read.

JOY--*I John 1:4&5--Real Joy is in fellowship with the Father and with His Son, Jesus Christ. Not in fellowship with others, even family, as pleasurable as that is.*

PEACE--*John 14:27--Jesus says, "Peace I leave with you, My peace I give unto you; not as the world giveth, give I unto you. Let not your heart be troubled, neither let it be afraid."*

HOPE--*Colossians 1:5a--"For the hope which is laid up for you in Heaven"--V27b--"Which is the Christ in you, the Hope of Glory."*

Early in December many organizations and churches came to the hospital visiting and bringing small gifts and cheer. Often they would bring carolers singing Christmas songs and carols.

Our hospital had hired two "recreation therapists" just out of college. They were delightful and such a help and encouragement to the children. When Melany had to lie flat on her back after myelograms and spinal taps, they came in and decorated the ceiling of her room and hung things on her bed frame. She was so pleased with them that she decided at ten that she wanted to be a "Play Person" when she grew up. That became her desire and later she went to college and majored in Therapeutic Recreation to pursue that dream.

As Christmas week came, the RTs were quite busy getting ready for a big party. The hospital had made a nice new well equipped Rec-Play Room. The girls had solicited gifts and food and entertainment for the children. There were about twenty five children on that floor, many of them cancer patients.

The party was scheduled for Dec. 24. This was their first big party however they did not realize that by Christmas Eve every child that had a hope of surviving a trip home had been allowed to go, even though many would return after Christmas Day.

Although Missy was in extreme pain with her back and joints she was really excited about the party. As one of the therapist pushed her wheel-chair down the hall she asked, "Why are all the rooms empty? Where are all the kids?"

My heart was sinking with each step. When we got to the playroom there was only one patient, his mother, and his sister. Herbie was a leukemia patient and was very sick, but he was there.

Missy's friend, Nancy, had come to join her. So we had four children, two mothers, many nurses and several doctors. It was a very sad time. Then the realization hit us, everyone that could, had gone home.

The recreation therapists played guitars and we all sang with large lumps in our throats. The doctors and nurses were very kind and tried to be jovial. One of the doctors told me later that he had cried all the way home and when he arrived he hugged his wife and children. He said that he had a real heart-felt appreciation for his healthy children. He added that it was different treating children in the hospital during the holidays and actually seeing the few that were left on Christmas Eve. Although he wasn't on call he came on Christmas Day and brought his children to see Melany. People were always so kind to us.

The party ended. The people left. Melany, Little Nancy and I went back to Melany's room. Herbie had only been able to stay a few minutes because he was so sick. Little Nancy's mother came and picked her up.

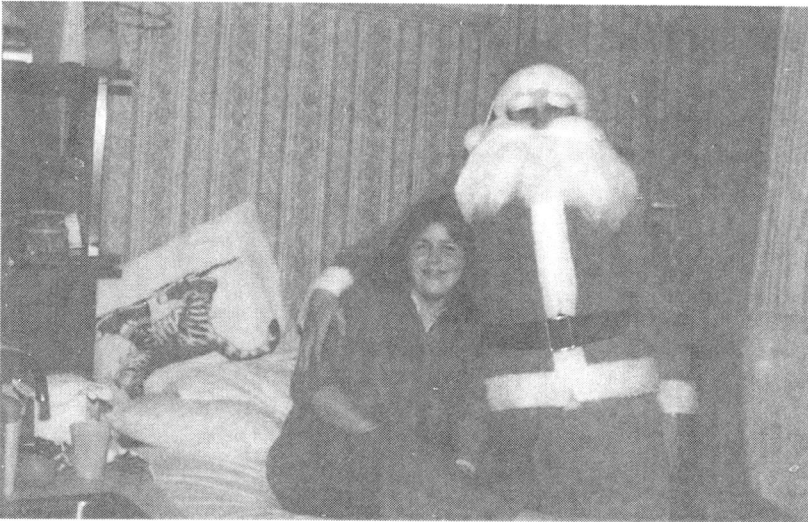

This was certainly going to be a different Christmas Eve and Christmas Day. Christmas Eve had always been very special at our house. My parents and James' parents always gathered with joy at my aunt's house. She and her husband had no children so they enjoyed ours immensely.

Through the years things changed. Both of our fathers had died but we still gathered and had a wonderful time. We knew that this year would be totally different. My uncle had died in

April and this would be a hard Christmas Eve and Christmas Day for my aunt.

James and Ric worked at a nuclear power plant. Ric had just started his first job. He was seventeen and was going to school to be an electrician like his father and his grandfather and was in a work training program. They were supposed to get off at five o'clock. The plans were they would pick up my mother-in-law, and then my mother and my aunt. The family was coming to the hospital to spend Christmas Eve with us. My aunt was fixing Christmas dinner for everyone the next day.

We had no idea just how different and difficult this Christmas Eve would be. At four thirty my husband called and said there was a big problem at work and he and our son could not leave. He said they would possibly have to work through the night.

My mother was in a wheelchair after suffering seven mini and two major strokes. She was staying with her sister while Melany was in the hospital. I called to tell them that James and Ric couldn't pick them up and to ask if my aunt could possibly bring my mother and pick up my mother-in-law.

Aunt Blanche said that it was very rainy and foggy and that she was afraid to drive. Also, that my mother was getting sick. They had already decided that she probably should not get out in the weather, nor did she need to be around Melany.

I tearfully called my mother-in-law. She had fixed some goodies to bring to the hospital. She was very disappointed at not getting to come.

I loved my mother-in-law dearly and it hurt me to think of her sitting all alone on Christmas Eve. I thought of my aunt caring for my mother and missing her dear husband, and of course, I missed my mother. I was born on Christmas Eve. We had been together each year except the two Christmases that she had to spend in the tuberculosis hospital in Rome (three hundred miles from our home in southwest Georgia) when I was six and seven years old.

I was becoming very teary although I was trying to be brave

in front of Missy. I cried, Missy cried then I said, "OK we are sad. We need to acknowledge that we are sad and find something to be thankful for."

We talked about how hard the two RTs had worked to make a nice party for two patients. One of them was driving home to her parents in Tennessee to-night, because she chose to stay and have the party although she could have left early.

We spoke of the doctors and nurses that gave of their time and came. Also, of all the people that had prepared and sent the goodies and favors. Then we prayed and thanked God for them and their families. Melany added, "And please keep their children healthy and happy."

We thanked God for our family and asked Him to be very near and dear to the grandmothers and aunt. We prayed for care and safety for our husband/dad and our brother/son. When we got through praying, Missy looked me straight in the eye and she asked, "How do you really think that we will do tonight?"

I didn't try to be light hearted or give clichés but simply and honestly said, "I really do not know. But I think we'll be OK because we have grateful hearts."

Things got very quiet on the floor with only two patients except those in the back in ICU. There were no happy voices or movements, no noises at all except a faint sound of Christmas Carols playing on the intercom in the hall.

Missy didn't even want the TV on. We were very reflective in our thoughts. About eight o'clock Melany asked me if I would go out to the waiting room and give her some time alone. This was a most unusual request from a ten year old on Christmas Eve.

I took my coat and told the nurse I was going on the porch. I stayed for almost an hour. I had always enjoyed the fifth floor porch, even in cold weather. It looked out over the parking lot, and a busy thoroughfare. There was a panoramic view of the city and the river beyond.

As I glanced at the fog encased parking lot, I was surprised that there were so few cars. No one chooses to be at the hospital on Christmas Eve unless it is necessary.

Even more amazing was the tripled-lane street in front of the hospital with very few cars. Everyone who had anywhere to go on Christmas Eve was already there with family or friends. How silent this night was. It must have been just like this the night that our Savior was born.

I felt so sad. I almost felt sorry for myself. I try to never allow myself this luxury because it can become a habit. I felt for each member of our family as we were always together at this time. We were painfully aware that each Christmas could be our last together and we tried to make each one special.

As I wept I thought of that first Christmas. How lonely Mary and Joseph must have been in that strange city. They had no family or friends there and no place to stay with a baby on the way.

How frightened they must have felt because of all that had happened in their lives. They surely had to face the uncertainty of their lives and of the future of their precious child. I felt that way too.

I thought of the stanza of "O Little Town of Bethlehem" that says, *"How silently, how silently the wondrous gift is given. So God imparts to human hearts, the blessing of His Heaven." It continues, "Where meek souls will receive Him still, the dear Christ enters in."*

Oh, how that silent, still, lonely frightened night for Mary and Joseph turned into the greatest event in Christian history. A child was born that brought Salvation, peace and eternal life to all generations if we will only accept Him as our Savior and Lord. This was a personal revelation for me, because of this event and this precious child, I can now face anything in life!

My heart was joyful and my step was light as I hurried back into Melany's room. Melany had already had her own quiet time and revelation. She said, "Mother, if we are really, truly celebrating Jesus' birthday in our hearts and lives, then it really doesn't matter where we are or if we are with people or alone." How very true, family and friends and traditions are nice and they bring happiness but they are not necessary for true joy.

We were much more content. All of a sudden, we heard a "Ho, ho, ho!" The door opened and there stood our dear, dear friends of many years, Joyce and Roy Scarborough. They were bringing gifts and Christmas cheer. We were so thrilled and so grateful that they had left their own family celebration to come spend this time with us. Our spirits were definitely lifted. We had a wonderful visit. After they left we thanked God for their willingness to give up time with their own family on Christmas Eve to come to the hospital with us. How grateful we were for all of our many friends. The few nurses that were there that night tried to be especially kind and jovial. As well as those that came on for the eleven-seven shift. One of those was a friend and a member of our church. Around midnight she came and called me out into the hall.

She said that a family was passing through Augusta in the early evening. They were going to visit their family in another town and had a serious accident. The father had died in the emergency room and they were bringing one child to intensive care, very seriously injured. One child was coming to the floor with less threatening injuries and the mother had only minor injuries. My friend said, "She desperately needs someone with her until family or friends can get here from out of town." She added that the hospital representative and the chaplain were with her now. "However," she continued, "I know that you have had much pain and heartache in your life and you have handled it well. This lady needs you." She said that she would stay with Melany as long as she could and that she would watch her closely if she went to sleep. She told me to come to the nurses' station as soon as I could, and the patient representative would take me to the lady.

As I was getting my clothes on I was really talking to the Lord. I said something to this effect, "Lord, I can't be a help for anyone tonight. You, and you alone, know how weak and weepy I am right now. Father, people have come to minister to me! How can I possibly help this lady with this great heartache?" I knew that I could only minister to her with God's help and grace.

That night I "relearned" four very valuable lessons that I had known through my own experience of pain:

FIRST, all this lady needed was for someone to just be there! She did not need an explicit explanation of thoughts, ideas or clichés. She just needed someone to say, "I'm here for you, and I care about your deep pain!" I simply was there and let her talk and cry, and at times just sit in reflective silence.

SECOND, that regardless of how bad our situations or circumstances seem, someone has greater troubles and pain than ours.

THIRD, we as individuals can unite our hearts in caring for others. Regardless of our race, religion (or lack of it) or socio-economic class. I was aware of this as others came forward to express their sympathy and care.

FOURTH, when we seek to help lessen the heart-aches of others, it helps to lessen our own.

As dawn neared, family members from their hometown about one hundred fifty miles away began arriving. Their priest came also. The lady had shared with me that she was a person of great faith.

I learned years ago that great faith is certainly necessary for our daily walk. However, it does not always take care of our deep present pain. Others, many in the name of our Heavenly Father, help us during this time until we are strong enough to return to our focus of our own faith.

After leaving my hospital room number I quietly slipped away. I returned to my own seemingly less painful situation. I was so thankful that I still had my husband, my son and my daughter, ill though she was.

This was one of numerous times in many hospitals that I was able to use my own heartache to help the hurting hearts of others.

We had already taken Melany to Medical College of Georgia, Emory, Children's Hospital, Duke, and Bowman Grey. They had all been helpful but no real diagnosis. Only the symptoms, apparent at the time were treated.

I really felt that God gave me a ministry and prepared me to help others (especially parents) that were hurting. In all of the hospitals there were so many hurting parents and grandparents. There were two scriptures that meant a lot to me and still do concerning this ministry:

First, *"To help (comfort) others by what you have been through (and God comforted you)"* II Corinthians 1:3&4.

Second, *"Therefore seeing we have this ministry, as we have received mercy, we faint not."* II Corinthians 4:1.

Christmas Day was a good day. Our family was there most of the day. Many friends came and some brought their children. Melany's close friend Susie Johnson came with her Dad, Dan. Sadly, the next Christmas Eve, Dan died at a young age of a heart attack. Some of Melany's friends from school and church came also. One of her doctors came and brought her an angel and the doctor that I mentioned earlier brought his children. Melany enjoyed them all although it was tiring for her.

After Melany died, I found her account of that first Christmas in the hospital. I remembered that she had shared it in some churches, encouraging people to remember those in the hospital, and how much a visit can help them cope with a difficult time. I want to share some of it with you. This is a ten year olds memories of that time.

The first part was much as I described it. She goes on to say, "When the party was over, I watched with a heavy heart as each of the doctors, nurses, therapists and friends left to go home to celebrate Christmas Eve with their families. How I longed to leave with them, so I could spend Christmas Eve at home with my family. The night before Christmas was always a very special time at our house. The entire family gathered and shared a meal. Then we read the Christmas Story and prayed before opening our presents. I was sure going to miss that. This was definitely going to be a very different Christmas Eve and Christmas Day for my whole family.

When I returned to my room after the party, I was glad for a quiet moment alone with my mom. I felt a little discouraged, so I asked, "Mom, we're going to be all alone on Christmas Eve Night. Do you think we can make it?"

She knelt by my wheelchair and with tears in her eyes replied, "I really don't know. During this time we will see whether we truly celebrate Christ's Birthday, like we claim, or whether we celebrate the tradition of family, friends and gifts that surrounds this holiday season. If we really celebrate Jesus Christ's Birthday, then we will have peace regardless of where we are, or what our circumstances may be; if not, we may fall apart."

Our dear friends, Joyce and Roy left their family to come and spend some time with me and Mom. They brought presents, but more important, they brought their presence.

After my visitors left later that night, I asked my mother to leave me alone for awhile, because I really needed to sort my thoughts. I thought about the Christmases I had spent in the past. I had been sick since I was seven years old, but I didn't allow this to hinder my joy of Christmas. I thought about the gifts I had received, the parades I went to, and my singing in the Christmas programs with my church choir. I thought about sitting by an open fire sharing a beautifully decorated tree with family and friends. I also thought about the joys of caroling and the visits I made to the hospitals trying to spread a little cheer. How ironic, here I was in the same hospital I had visited; however, now I found myself alone and cheerless.

I have never questioned the Lord (and I have always tried not to complain) about the progressing neuro-muscular disease that has robbed me of my ability to walk and caused limited use of one hand and constant pain over most of my body. It had already placed me in the hospital over thirty-five times, denying me many things that I have really enjoyed.

As I laid my heart open before the Lord, I said, "Lord, you have blessed me with many things, you have given me real peace even during these difficult days. But Lord, every tradition of Christmas Eve that I've held dear you've allowed to be taken from me this year. Lord, I'm humbly seeking the real meaning of Christmas, please help me see it."

I thought about some of the joys and gifts that I had already witnessed. They came in strange packages, but they were worth receiving. I thought about the Recreational Therapists that cared enough to provide a lovely party for one patient. I thought about the doctors who took time off from their busy schedules to attend the party and blend their voices in singing. I thought of one of my own doctors, who came even though it was his day off. I remembered the tears that I saw in his eyes as he hugged me good-bye, showing that he really cared. I thought of the nurses that went out of their way to be loving and cheerful, even though I'm sure they longed to be with their families. I remembered my pastor and youth director who visited me so faithfully.

As I continued to think, my mind wandered to the carolers who gave of their time to help cheer me, just as I had done at one time. I knew the Lord blessed me with very special friends who visited me during these busy days of preparation (Many others came on Christmas Day). My thoughts turned to our special family friends, Joyce and Roy, who left their family celebration to come to see us because they couldn't stand the thought of mother and me being alone.

In the stillness of the night, I picked up my Bible and re-read the beautiful story of the first Christmas. I felt excited as I experienced a thrill of new discoveries in my reading and meditations. I'd never before been this still and quiet on

Christmas Eve. I realized I'd never been so totally aware of Christ's wondrous birth, his selfless life, or his deep love for me that compelled him to die on the cruel cross. I was so thankful that he arose victorious, promising me eternal life.

Suddenly, I realized, I was really experiencing peace and joy. Now, more than ever before, I understood the true meaning of Christmas.

"A season in the rain will end at last,
A season full of pain will surely pass.
The reason will be plain someday,
When love reveals its goal
Such are the seasons of the soul."
Lee Ezell
Find Hope When Life Is Not Fair

"Our best hopes and dreams for our children pale in comparison
to those God has for them."
Parenting the Way God Parents

"HE WHO SUFFERS MOST HAS MOST TO GIVE."
Streams In the Desert

CHAPTER IV
<u>PRAYER SUPPORT</u>

"When thou passeth through the waters, they shall never overflow." Isaiah 43:2

"We know not what we should pray for."
Romans 8:26

As stated earlier all children need discipline, including disabled ones. As Melany got sicker we prayed sincerely that God would guide us to help her keep her sweet spirit and follow in His ways.

Melany's pain started around age seven and we changed our methods of discipline.

We had tried to use spanking (meaning a few swats on the area that God had padded well) as a very last resort. We tried talking first (they hated that) before using a minute in time out for each year of age. Ric seldom got to the spanking stage.

When we tried talking, Melany would put her fingers in her ears. She would shake her head back and forth and repeat several times, "Don't tell me those words, just spank me and get through with it."

When placed in timeout she would say, "You can make me sit down but I'm still standing up on the inside."

James believed he was too big to hit little people and never spanked the children. I surely did not have the heart to inflict more pain on Missy even a light reminder of a swat.

All children have errant qualities sometimes. Melany was a very loving child with a sweet spirit but she too had her moments. We knew the Bible says in Proverbs 22:15a, *"Foolishness is bound in the heart of a child."* We prayed diligently that God would help remove the foolishness from her heart and life.

Later as preteens and teenagers we would restrict a privilege. The one most hated was writing a thoughtful page on the misbehavior in question. We did not use this if Melany's hands were swollen or painful. It was hard to restrict a privilege when she had so few.

Melany endured many months of pain including her Christmas stay and was finally able to leave the hospital. The doctors were still treating the symptoms of her disease that had not yet been identified. She would improve for a while then become very ill again. The pain in her back never eased completely.

After much prayer from many sources our doctors finally diagnosed a "contained" viral infection in her spinal column. After treatment she improved but they knew this was not her only problem.

Missy kept up her school work during her hospitalization. The wonderful teachers brought assignments by the hospital. She would complete them and take tests when she was able. After returning home she loved attending school even part time.

We received prayer support for years from family, friends and people we never met. We received cards and letters from many churches including our own church family assuring us of their prayer support for Melany and for us. It became evident to me in the summer Missy was ten years old how important the prayers of intercession can be to others.

The doctors sent us to the famed Johns Hopkins Hospital in Baltimore, Maryland. James stayed home because he was paid by the hour and we had spent much time and money traveling to different hospitals in the past few years.

Ric was seventeen and was delighted to help drive the five hundred miles. We went a few days early before our scheduled appointment and visited our dear friends originally from Augusta. Jo and Jim Gregory were now living in Laurel,

Maryland, between Washington, D.C., and Baltimore. We enjoyed many times of fellowship and sightseeing with Jo and Jim while we lived there when Ric was two years old.

During the three days we were in Laurel Melany was able to do some sightseeing. We went to Washington and to her delight saw the president's motorcade. We also went to the new port and marina in Baltimore. Although she was unable to walk far and used a wheelchair she enjoyed it immensely. She especially liked the little ice cream shop that overlooked the Chesapeake Bay and our visit to the quaint little town of Ellicott City, Maryland.

At Johns Hopkins there were days of extensive painful tests including many she had previously endured. I often told her, "Remember, nothing lasts forever, just think-'This will soon be over.'" But it was hard for her and for us.

We finally received the diagnosis, of Behcet's Disease often called Behcet's Syndrome. It is very rare and usually affects adolescent boys in Middle Eastern Countries and Central Asia.

The only printed information they gave us was two pages lifted out of a medical book. That was thirty two years ago but today they have volumes of information available plus the internet.

When the studies were completed Ric and I were taken into a conference room where several doctors were sitting around a long oval table. They were very kind and caring as they each shared from their specialty fields and their knowledge and perspective about the disease. They had studied and were all very informed about Behcet's.

They said that it is a devastating disease. They put it in layman's terms and described it as being similar to multiple sclerosis. MS attacks the skeletal muscles as does Behcet's. Behcet's also attacks the smooth muscles such as heart, lungs, supporting muscles and neurological tissues. The disease would have times of great intensity as it literally could go from part to part of her body or from organ to organ. They continued saying there was no cure for it at that time and the medicines available could not be used with her because her heart was already affected.

Their consensus was her doctors in Augusta would only be able to treat the symptoms as they appeared, with steroids and other remedies as they became available. Their opinion was that the doctors were already treating her correctly. The prognosis was she would live approximately five years if the disease progressed rapidly and possibly ten years if it progressed slowly.

In stunned silence Ric and I listened as the doctors shared briefly with us from their notes.

The cardiologist said her heart is already effected as at times it would beat up to one hundred sixty to one hundred eighty beats per minute. He said that this is probably what would take her life. Her doctor at home already had given her the right medicine which was not always effective.

She had episodes of tachycardia as long as she lived. However they were right, in the end her precious little heart just gave out.

The ophthalmologist said it would probably effect her eyesight at some point and could possibly lead to blindness. Her eyesight remained fine but she had a visual problem for about a year after she had a "vascular incident." She had a "beam" in the center of her vision of her right eye. Later it was like looking through a "screen," before it finally disappeared. There was no treatment which was very frustrating but she handled it like she did everything else she just went on doing the best she could and never complained.

The pulmonary specialist said her lungs would probably be affected and she would possibly have to use oxygen. She had to start using oxygen when she was eighteen and had a non-invasive respirator two years before her death.

The orthopedist and rheumatologist shared information about her joints and bones. She suffered with joint and muscle pain for years. The nephrologist told of possible kidney involvement. She did not have that until the last year of her life.

The urologist explained what had happened with the bladder and the urethra and the ulcers that were present. He said that would continue.

The gastroenterologist also commented on what had already happened to her intestines and her bowels. Through the years she had twenty surgeries and many surgical procedures on her stomach and intestines. She had a colostomy for ten years and an ileostomy for the last ten years.

The neurologist explained the neuromuscular problems and of the brain cell function. She had all of those for many years.

The vascular doctor told us this disease often produced aneurysms and embolisms. Melany had many blood clots and was on heparin drip for about six years before she died.

Finally the unbelievable came from the gynecologist. His findings were that there was already a lot of scar tissue in her reproductive organs and she was beginning to have signs of a form of endometriosis. He felt she should have surgery or she would continue having severe infections. He said with any neurological disease a person could become sepsis (a severe infection that gets into the blood stream), very quickly.
The surgery could be done there or at home but it needed to be done soon. He gave me papers to read and sign if we wanted to have it there.

The internist, who seemed to lead the discussion asked if we had any questions. I remember feeling for the first time in my life I was surely going to faint. I started to cry and weakly asked, "Are you absolutely sure that this is what she has?"

The internist replied that they were sure. Then he continued, "We are so sorry to have to tell you this, and so sorry that at this time in this great institution we are unable to help her or to offer you much hope."

I felt completely numb all over. Ric spoke up and asked if they would contact us in the future if they found something that would help her.

The facilitator replied, "All the doctors here today will send transcripts back to Augusta with you to help the doctors and we will be available for consultation as the disease progresses and perhaps one day we will know more about it." Then they all left the room.

The chaplain came in and prayed with us and asked if there was anything he could do. We thanked him and he left his card.

Ric and I sat in disbelief and talked briefly. We had brought a child here praying and believing we would get help for painful ulcers and swollen feet and hands. Now they were talking about possibly removing the reproductive organs of a ten year old who loved little babies.

I knew her daddy was waiting eagerly by the phone for the results of the consultation. I dreaded having to tell him they could not help her. Also, that she was headed for five to ten years of pain and devastation and then would probably die. I also dreaded the fact I had to go into Melany's room with a cheery heart and face and talk to her.

I said to Ric, "I don't know what we need now except the Lord." Then we went to the chapel to pray.

I was so burdened and scared I did not know at that moment how to pray or what to pray for. I remembered Lee Gibbs (my former Sunday School Teacher) sharing with us how once when her little Tony almost died she could simply utter groanings to the Holy Spirit in prayer. I murmured something like this "Oh precious Holy Spirit take my prayer and purify it to the Father for His will to be done and for His answer to our situation. In the precious name of Jesus Christ my Lord and Savior. Amen."

Ric said "Mom, go somewhere and get yourself together. I'll go play a board game with Mimi until you return." I must have been in bad shape for a seventeen year old boy to notice.

I needed some things from my car at the very top of the parking deck. I stood for a long time trying to process all that I had heard and looking at the beautiful skyline of Baltimore.

Dusk has always been my favorite time of the day. I watched as the lights started coming on over the city. I could see a church and a cathedral, suddenly I felt such a calm and peace as I realized it was Wednesday night and I knew many people were praying for us. What a comfort!

When I entered Melany's room she and her brother were playing and laughing. I started to tell her the visual reminder of God's care I had just experienced but she stopped me. She told us the doctor had come and said they were probably going to do some surgery on her tomorrow morning and he would be back later.

She said, "I cried because I wanted to go home."

"When my supper tray came and I saw that it was Wednesday and, Momma, people at home and other places are praying for me tonight so it's going to be OK!"

I called James and told him all the doctors had said and what we were facing the next day. For a brief time he was so choked up he could not speak, then we cried together. I told him about my roof top experience and Melany's hospital room experience.

In his wonderful calm way, James reminded me as he has done many times, "Sweet, we must have faith and not run ahead of God." I always felt better when I talked to him, even six hundred miles away.

When I had talked with Ric, and then with James on the phone we all agreed that we would not tell Melany any of this. We simply would tell her that the doctors at home were treating her correctly. We watched in great horror for years as all the doctors told us came to pass. When she was much older she read about the disease but by then she had already experienced most of it. She still had faith that she would be healed.

James and I had many phone conversations during the next few days. James was so burdened by her prognosis he said to me, "Tell Missy for the first time ever [I doubted that] I am going to "pull rank" on Mom. Tell her I have reconsidered and you can take her and get her little ears pierced when she gets home."

I agreed she needed something special to happen for her and so did her dad. Ric thought it was a good idea too.

When told what her dad said, she replied, "No, I don't want to do that now. I want to have something to look forward to when I am thirteen."

About nine o'clock as I came from the phone booth into the waiting room I saw a couple sitting there. I sat down to dry my eyes and get myself composed before going back into Melany's room.

We started talking and I learned they lived in Baltimore and had come to visit their grand-Daughter who was scheduled for a tonsillectomy and ear surgery the next morning. I introduced myself and told them I was from Augusta, Georgia. The man said, "Did you say Wiggins?" I nodded and they looked at each other as the gentleman (Mr. Atkins) pulled a paper from his pocket. He said, "When we prayed for our grand-daughter a few minutes ago in our church we prayed for a little girl in this hospital named Melany (he pronounced it Ma-laney, but that was fine) Wiggins from Augusta, Georgia.

We learned later that on Tuesday our friends in Laurel, had asked their neighbors to include Melany on the prayer list at their church. The neighbor had called her sister in Baltimore and asked to have her Methodist Church family to pray. Mr. Atkins asked if they could go in and pray with Melany.

Isn't God good!! He had given me peace on the roof of the parking garage that whatever happened He was in control. He gave Melany the assurance people were praying for her and everything would be alright. Then He sent a messenger to reaffirm the prayers of God's people.

We should never underestimate the power of the prayers that we pray in intercession for others. It may be their life line at that very time.

It is wonderful when we get affirmation of our faith. But many times we have to trust and believe without any outward sign--this is true faith. Non-Christians or Christians who are not walking close to God do not understand this kind of faith. We should not judge them, only pray for them because the first part of I Corinthians 2:14 says, *"But the natural man receiveth not the things of the Spirit of God; for they are foolishness unto him."*

Melany did not have the surgery there and her doctor in Augusta treated her and was able to do a less drastic procedure.

James and I had faced everything in our life with care and faith. This was the only time we were almost in complete denial. As we read and reread the information we had been given about Behcet's we just could not believe it. We would read the papers and pray over them asking God to please let this diagnosis be wrong. We went back to the local doctors who had received the information from Johns Hopkins, they all confirmed it was true, they agreed that was the correct diagnosis. One of the doctors at the Medical College of Georgia showed us previous notes where they had suspected Behcet's, which was one reason they had wanted us to take her to Johns Hopkins. He said, "We see horses, they see zebras." He also said they did not want to tell us this until they were certain.

The doctors now knew what they were dealing with, and they would continue to treat it as best they could. Years later Melany's pediatrician told us that he had been able to identify two other cases of Behcet's because of the information he had learned from Melany's case. He said it was difficult to diagnose because of the myriad symptoms that came at different times. It was like putting a puzzle together.

We had to accept the reality of what was happening and be thankful for finally getting the diagnosis. We thanked God everyday for the wonderful doctors that had worked so diligently trying to help Missy, and asked for continued guidance for them.

We had a small card that simply said,

"Believe in the sun when it doesn't shine,
And God when He is silent."

We continued depending on God and on daily prayer support from our friends, family and Prayer Warriors that prayed everyday for us.

Is there some earnest prayers unanswered yet,
Or answered not as you had thought it would be?
God will make clear His purpose by-and-by.
He keeps the key.
And of the door of all thy future life,
He keeps the key.
Unfailing comfort, sweet and blessed rest,
To know of EVERY door
He keeps the key,
Then He at last when just HE sees 'tis best,
Will give it to THEE.
Anonymous
STREAMS IN THE DESERT

"Our children learn to have a heart for those in need when there is an atmosphere of kindness and willingness to help each other in our homes."
Parenting the Way God PARENTS

CHAPTER V
PRAYER SUSTAINING

"Men ought always to pray," Luke 18:1
"Make thy petition deep." Isaiah 7:11

Through the years we learned what it means to continually be sustained in and through prayer. The teachers and school staff were always understanding and so helpful.

Melany studied very diligently. I would go everyday for her school work. She would complete it as she could and we would return it to be graded. The teachers continued to come to the house and hospital to help her and give tests. They willingly gave so much of their time and went far above any call of duty.

Mimi continued to love school and enjoyed the social aspect as well and was able to take a few class trips. How thankful I was and still am for the teachers and students that went the "extra mile" to include her.

She never asked, "Why me?" nor did she complain about things she was unable to do. I know many times her heart hurt just as ours did for the things she missed.

During her freshman year of high school she was using a small scooter to get around and we purchased a van to transport the scooter. She still could walk some and use crutches in the house and in the classroom.

Melany had planned to go with her class on a three day trip. We had taken her large suitcase to the school the evening before so they could pack early and leave at eight o'clock the following morning. They were to leave an open space for her scooter to fit in.

It was obvious during the night she would not be able to go.

We had called one of our faithful physicians about seven a.m. and he said to meet him at the emergency room around eight-thirty.

We called and told the teachers not to load her bags. Melany wanted to go to school with me to pick up her suitcase and see the class leave. They put her suitcase in the back and many of her classmates came to the van because she was too ill to get out. They hugged her and told her how sorry they were she could not join them.

After the bus was loaded she asked me to wait and as it pulled away I looked over at Melany, big tears were silently rolling down her cheeks but she didn't say a word. I embraced her and we cried together. Finally she said, "Let's pray now that they have a safe trip and a very enjoyable time," and we did just that.

On the way to the hospital Melany shared her remembrances of the trips she had been a part of. Her best memory by far was a trip to Disney World. The headmaster, Arvil Holt, and his wife (Melany's teacher), Gerry, had offered to be responsible for Melany. I couldn't go on the school trip because my Mother had suffered a massive stroke and was in intensive care not expected to live.

Melany had thoroughly enjoyed the trip. I'm not sure about the Holt's. They had assumed a mammoth responsibility. They probably never knew what it had really meant to Melany, as well to James and me, for their goodness to her. All of the school staff had always gone above the call of duty to help Melany.

When we reached the hospital, the doctor admitted her to the hospital and she stayed for a month.

Melany was able to go on several trips through the years. She was very mission minded and had completed all the steps in Girls in Action and Acteens. She received the highest recognition as Queen Regent with a Scepter in Service (photo, next page).

Melany had wanted to be a missionary, so one of the highlights in her life was the mission trips that she went on, especially the one to Kansas. She also made another trip to the

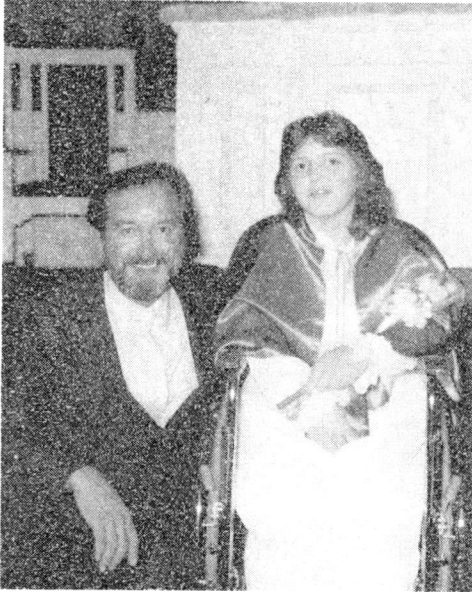

Acteen Convention in Fort Worth, Texas. She was able to go on one choir tour across the states of North Carolina and Tennessee where they attended the World's Fair. Melany always rode the bus with the others. I drove our van in case she had an emergency. She did have a few but that was her everyday life.

Although we tried to keep things as "normal" as possible for the family. I realized just how different our lives had to be. When we arrived in the different towns on church trips or with friends on vacations, the other ladies would be looking for the malls and outlet stores for shopping. I was looking for hospital signs that pointed to the hospitals, and how far they were from where we were staying. Several times we did have to go the hospital.

Several summers we were blessed to be able to go to our Baptist Center at Ridgecrest, North Carolina for music week. That was always enjoyable, usually there were seven to ten ladies (all close friends) and fifteen to twenty children and young people. The young children went to a musical day camp with all the amenities. The older ones and teenagers went to

Centrifuge where they had music and a wonderful time. I took classes in writing and hymn writing and missions. Missy and I really looked forward to these trips.

As Missy's condition declined she was hospitalized many times. She was in the hospital for several months, through another Christmas, when she was thirteen. We had added a new wonderful doctor, Dr. Richard Magruder, a Rheumatologist.
The first time Melany saw him she said, "Mother, he is the kindest, most gentle doctor that I have ever seen." She had seen many and liked them all but she loved him dearly and prayed for him even after he retired from his practice.

During this long hospital stay Missy completely lost all walking ability even though they did physical therapy to keep her muscles as strong and pliable as possible. She was unable to balance herself even when held upright.

The doctors finally felt they had done all they could do for her condition and we could take her home in a wheelchair.

This was before we knew much about home health care. They sent me to a medical store for a wheelchair for her. I purchased one that was really too large and bulky for a thirteen year old. In the large hospital rooms, with wide halls and bathrooms it was easy to maneuver a wheelchair, but it was not quite that easy at home.

James and Ric rearranged the furniture in Missy's bedroom and we took her home. As we rolled the wheelchair into the living room I thanked God our house was flat on a concrete slab and required no ramp.

We took Melany into her pretty white and gold bedroom that she hadn't seen for a year. She was very happy. She looked into her closet at the new clothes we had bought last year with the tags still attached. We were all so thankful she had come home again.

Missy needed to go to the bathroom and reality hit. Ric pushed her wheelchair to the bathroom door but it was not wide enough to go through. Missy started crying as James, Ric and I encircled her and we all cried. We ALL had the same thought, James or Ric could get her into the bathroom today but what would I do tomorrow when they went back to work?

Her dad lifted her up and took her into the bathroom and I helped her. Later we widened the bathroom door. He returned her to the chair and pushed her into the living room where our family had an "attitude conference," this was one of many.

My stable husband was a man of few words, but usually wise ones. I will never forget what he said to her and to us. He said, "Missy, we have taken you to five of the best teaching hospitals in our nation. They were not able to offer us any help we cannot get here at home. Your caring doctors tell us that you will never be able to walk again. I would give my last cent and last breath if you could be well again but unless God chooses to heal you, and He can, we must all live with this situation.

We cannot choose what happens to us in life, but we can choose how we handle it. We will all have to work on our attitudes. Every time Ric, or your mother or I see a strong healthy child, we must thank God for that child. We cannot dwell on the fact that you no longer have their abilities. This will not be easy for us or for you.

You must work especially hard not to let your heart and mind become angry and bitter over things you can no longer do or can't control. For I would truly rather you have a crippled body than a crippled mind and heart."

I thought of these wise words many times as I stood at the window watching the neighborhood children running and playing. I watched with tears as they were gleefully going to school while my child languished on her bed in pain. When the youth choir sang at church, I was painfully reminded how much she enjoyed singing, playing the piano, the guitar, the hand bells and the glockenspiel. She was slowly losing the use of her hands and her coordination was not good. These days of musical delight would probably be no more for her enjoyment.

I did learn to look at each precious child and audibly thank

God for their abilities. I prayed they would be kept from physical harm and disease. I prayed for their parents and that they would appreciate the healthy children that they had. This attitude continues to-day many years later and has gotten me through many trying days!

In this book I may have overstated several times that Melany never complained or asked of God or us, "Why did this happen to me?" or "Why can't I?" It was very true, although I'm sure there were times that she felt this inside of her heart. She just dealt with it and never expressed it to others, unless it was appropriately with counselors.

I know she was often "reflective." I remember one particular time that happened the second year after she was in a wheelchair full time. In the fall, James, Melany and I went to the mountains for our "annual" (when Melany was able), trip to see the beautiful fall leaves. We always went with our longtime friends, the Hattaways.

We visited the Toccoa Falls in North Georgia. The falls are very high with a path that leads almost to the top. As we sat on the benches in the little park at the foot of the falls, Melany started sharing with us. James and I had already heard part of what she was telling, from our youth director and some of the counselors that had accompanied the young people to "Youth Camp," held there each year.

Melany gave a humorous and detailed account of her last visit there, the summer before her lengthy stay when she had been confined to the wheelchair. We all listened as she reminisced how she had led the "Jericho March" up to the top of the falls. They had to stop several times at the little rest areas along the way. She joyfully shared how great it was, laughing about various little snippets that occurred along the way. She recalled that about half way up, she just gave out of energy (she was on crutches). The wonderful young men in the group took turns and formed a "human chair," by twos interlocking their arms and carrying her the rest of the way. She finished by adding "Friends are always so good to me, and so are others."

She became quiet and somewhat wistfully asked us to just let her sit there alone for a little while and think of how wonderful her life had been. June, Tony and I went into the little shop there, and Tony kept a watchful eye on Melany, in case she needed us. James and Bill left to go down to the little country store. When Melany motioned for us to come out, they came back with several lengths of rope.

Melany still seemed very reflective, but she was delighted as they secured the ropes to the front, back and sides of her wheelchair. They slowly pulled her up the path, gladly stopping at the little rest areas along the way. I made pictures as they neared the highest place they were allowed to go.

After enjoying the view, and taking a well deserved rest, they started down. Then they discovered that it was much more difficult than the laborious climb had been. The people that had gathered in the little park area to observe the feat, had made several comments about how they could get her down. A couple had stated they thought it was dangerous to take her up. I think we all agreed with that statement, but we were used to Melany's life being a little dangerous, she thought it was adventurous.

The men had tried bringing the wheelchair down backward, so she would not fall out. Finally, they just stopped, and sent Tony down to have June and me to call security and ask for some help. Four of the young college men were there with us. They immediately started the climb, and as we all watched, they formed a human chain, and slowly and methodically began to bring her down.

The crowd cheered and applauded, June and I prayed very diligently. Just as they safely reached the bottom of the path, Melany used one of her much expressed cliques, "The Lord always sends angels when I need help, they're just not usually this good looking." The profusely sweating, short of breathe, grateful Dads thanked the students and offered a monetary thanks. Then James led the entire group in a grateful prayer of thanksgiving for God's care and for all who had assisted and those who supported the efforts.

The young students refused the gratuity but they did go with us to a little café down the road for lunch. We had a very enjoyable time. I've often wondered where these fine young men are now. Two planned to go into the ministry, one was interested in music, the third was not sure, he said it would not be in difficult rescues, he was not strong enough. We all laughed, they were all delightful.

As we all expressed our embarrassment yet thankfulness that the security had arrived just as they came down with Melany safely in tow. They brought with them the firetruck, police and an ambulance Melany said that we always had to create a disturbance. Her dad was grateful that none of them reprimanded the two "old men," for trying such a ridiculous undertaking.

Prayer sustained our family through the high school years. Melany always maintained a good attitude but occasionally my good attitude was tested and had to be readjusted.

Melany was in the hospital for her sixteenth birthday. She was in a lot of pain and had just come out of intensive care. They had removed a large part of her colon a few days earlier. She could not eat but asked me to bring her cake and cupcakes to the hospital to share with the doctors, nurses and staff. We had done this at least twice before as we celebrated her birthday in the hospital. I had ordered a small birthday cake with an angel on the top and six dozen cupcakes. I knew from past experience that people from all over the hospital would come by her room.

I had arrived at the bakery around eleven thirty am. I thought that folks would stop by after their lunch break. The bakery was crowded and the lady in front of me was highly irate. She was screaming at the poor saleslady and demanded to see the owner. The owner came out and apologized for the mistake they had made and she offered the birthday cake for free.

The lady would have no consolation. She continued ranting, "You don't understand, I am taking this cake to school for my child's eighth birthday party. She wanted a cake with a ballerina in a blue tutu and slippers and blue flowers, not pink.

"I don't have time for you to correct your mistake. You have completely ruined my daughter's eighth birthday and my day as well." She snatched the cake and abruptly left leaving the owner and saleslady very embarrassed and apologetic.

I paid for my cake and cupcakes and left. I sat for a while in my car and wept. I said, "Oh Lord, how full of trivia that lady is. She's completely unglued by a pink ballerina instead of a blue one. How will she ever teach her daughter to deal with the real disappointments of life? She should be so grateful to have a healthy child and be able to celebrate her birthday with friends and classmates. I'm simply praying that my child lives until I get back to the hospital, and Lord, I am thankful that you have spared her life this long for this birthday. Lord, the world is so full of trivia, and my heart is so full of pain!"

The Lord reminded me gently that when my life is going well that I too become involved in trivia. When that happens I'm not as aware of other people's needs either. I still pray every day in my quiet time, "Lord, please keep my heart tender, my spirit kind and my mind aware of other's needs."

The Lord helped me to readjust my thoughts and my attitude. I have to do this quite often with the Lord's help, I surely cannot do it on my own.

Prayer sustained our family through Melany's high school years. We always appreciated so very much the wonderful attitudes of her classmates and friends.

There was a group of young boys that carried her in her wheelchair to the third floor of our church anytime that she was able to attend "Joy Explosion" on Wednesday nights. We always told her friends and their families that if there was an accident of any kind, we would not blame them, and we didn't believe in suing. We felt that they were as careful with her as they could be. We did not want them to feel guilty if there was an accident.

On Wednesday evenings after Prayer Meeting and Joy Explosion the young people gathered in the gym and played games, including volley ball or basketball. One of them would wheel Missy around when it was her turn. Often, they would almost sling her out of her wheelchair.

The mothers watched this, and would become very nervous and would express to me they could not believe that I allowed it. James and I explained to them how important it was for her to be included in the things the young people did. We and Melany, had rather her be included and hurt a little physically than to be hurt emotionally. We felt when you are over-protective with disabled children or adults, it makes other people uncomfortable and they withdraw from them. Physical pain will heal, but often emotional pain does not.

Her peers were very protective of her. The photographer who made the senior class picture on the lower steps of our church thought the wheelchair was a big distraction. In his young unthinking manner he asked if Melany could stand long enough for the picture to be made so that the wheelchair would not ruin the picture.

Her teacher said that the boys and girls verbally attacked the poor guy. They told him she had been a part of their class for twelve years and they loved her, wheelchair and all. They continued that there was nothing she could do that would ruin their picture. In fact they said it would be ruined if she wasn't in it.

The teacher said that the poor fellow was so embarrassed that he apologized many times. He felt so bad that he went to the trouble to get Melany's address and write her a note of apology.

With a sense of humor Melany educated many people in dealing with disabilities.

She smiled sweetly as people talked over her head or turned

their backs in a crowd and ignored her. Our family and most of our friends either sit down or kneel whenever possible to talk to anyone in a wheelchair.

Missy laughed repeatedly as a sales clerk asked the person with her what she needed, or what they could do for her. We tried to nicely say, "Just ask her." However, she was less amused when the checkout person gave her change to me or a friend with her. Once it was given to a total stranger standing behind her.

At counters they would look over her head and serve the person behind her. Even with the disabilities act the public still has a lot to learn about disabled people and their needs. Most disabled people just take it in stride, although at times it does hurt.

Melany's classmates were so considerate of her. Every Christmas if she was unable to attend the Christmas Party at school they brought the party to her, whether at home or in the hospital. They were always welcomed in our home and came often.

When they were planning the Junior-Senior Party (both years) two of her friends, Kevin and Barry, went to the places where they were to be held ahead of time, to be sure that they could get Melany in comfortably. What wonderful forethought for two seventeen year old boys!

Melany was able to attend the Junior-Senior both years. What a wonderful time she had. What a difficult time we had finding a pretty gown that wouldn't entangle with the wheels on her chair.

The wonderful night of graduation finally arrived. We have large families and many members came from out of town plus many friends.

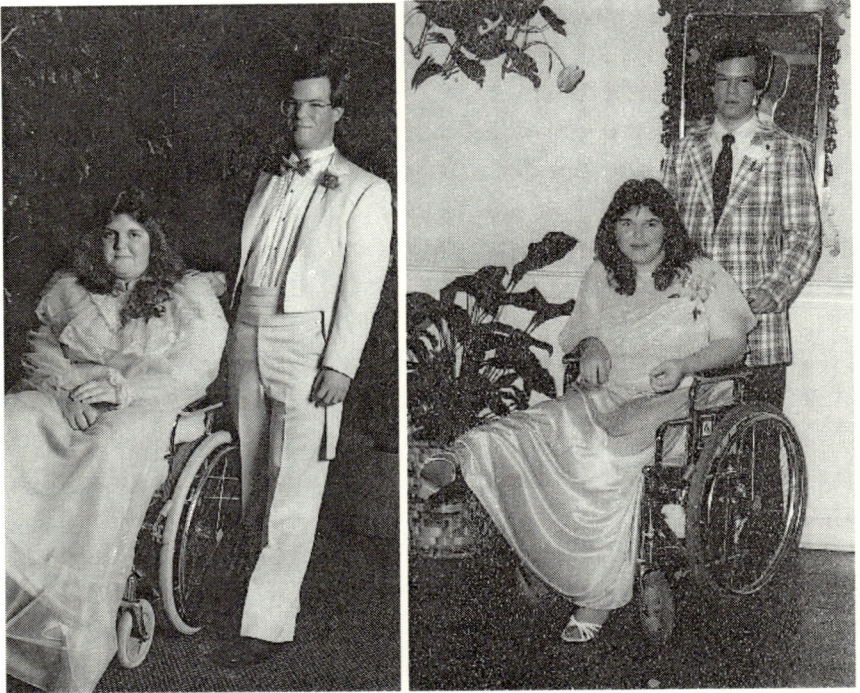

Melany and Tony, 1984 (left) and 1985

Melany had never made any grade below an A all through twelve grades. She was the valedictorian and made a touching speech. I am including it here, because so many people have asked for a copy and many others said that it was so very thought-provoking for them.

May 26, 1985

Classmates, faculty, parents and honored guests:

This is one of the happiest days of my life, and it a real honor for me to speak to you tonight. If I could ask each one of you here tonight one question, "What is the greatest need in your life?" most would give the same answer--happiness or peace.

I would like for us to think briefly on this--

The dictionary describes happiness as "The quality or state of being happy; good fortune, pleasure, contentment; joy!" It's quite simple to describe, yet very hard to find.

Some think success in life brings happiness--yet more people who have acquired success visit psychologists than another group of people.

Most people believe money will surely bring happiness but many suicides and attempted suicides are reported among the wealthy.

For some, finding the right mate would certainly bring happiness though statistics tell us that approximately half of all marriages will end in divorce.

We, as young people, often feel that finishing high school and perhaps going on to college, and getting out from under parental authority will definitely bring happiness. And yet our future is uncertain. It is a little frightening and we really fear failure in life.

Many feel that good health would surely make one happy--yet some of the most miserable people we know have a strong body and a great measure of health.

I would like to share some thoughts of some simple things in which I find happiness, and I encourage you to make your own list. REMEMBER--happiness is receiving and being able to give to others.

To me, happiness is first of all knowing Christ as my Savior, being assured that He has prepared a home for me in Heaven, and being able to claim all of His promises made in the Bible. Also, knowing that God has and will sustain me through every difficult situation in my life.

Happiness is being able to give my life and my all back to the Lord.

My parents once gave me a plaque that hangs on my wall. You may be familiar with the verse--"What you are is God's gift to you--What you become is your gift to God!"

Happiness is having a church family that loves and supports me, that prays for me and other young people, as well as those in need. Having a pastor and staff that often remember me with cards, letters, visits and prayers.

It was members of my church family--Mr. Melvin Barton and Mr. Leon Barton that donated the material for a ramp my dad and Mr. McManus built to get me into the junior high building. It was Mr. Don Cheeks who helped my parents make my high school education possible and I deeply appreciate these men and others who encouraged me.

Happiness is knowing and studying under some of the finest teachers anywhere! As I look at this group of teachers--starting with

Mrs. McKnight in kindergarten and dear Mrs. Sapp in first grade, whom we honored today, all through the years you have enlightened and encouraged me. Without your dedication and especially the junior and senior high school teachers I've had for the past six years--I would never have made it. Some of you helped me after school, at lunch, during your free periods, and even at home or the hospital. All of you went above and beyond the call of duty--including the principal, counselor, and secretaries. I hope that I have personally thanked each one of you--but tonight especially, I would like to say a great big THANK YOU!

Happiness is being surrounded by friends. My life, like many of yours has not always been easy, yet you as friends (especially my peers) have helped me far more that you will ever know. Leslie, Andrea and Tricia, willingly shared their notes with me when I was unable to attend classes. The guys were always there to help get me in or out of wherever I needed to go. You'll never know how you brightened my day with a phone call, or offering to take me to the mall or a movie, or coming by for a visit or simply slowing your pace, so I could keep up. Many of you have allowed me to give back to you my thoughts, ideas, prayers, help, and encouragement during your hard times and I appreciate this as well.

Happiness to me is having good doctors, nurses and therapists. Now this may seem strange to some of you, to be happy about a doctor (especially when you get his bill!) but over the years, these people have become a vital part of my life--They are so good to me. I pray for them every day. I appreciate their dedication and care for all of us.

I thank the Lord for the opportunity to live in a country where quality medical help is so readily available.

Happiness is being a part of a loving family. Never one day in my life have I not felt total unconditional love from my family. We are fun-loving (as most of you know). We laugh a lot and have a lot of good times together!

My parents led me to the Lord when I was a young child. My mother taught me that nothing in life could ever happen to me that our loving Heavenly Father did not allow and have control of. She said that if He allowed something to be taken from my life (and this applies to all of you as well) that He would certainly replace it with more. She taught me to look for and expect the "MORES" in life--and I have found many.

My dad told me when I was first confined to a wheel chair that I could not control what happened to my mind and heart. And, that if I let bitterness, anger and jealously (over what others could do or have, or be), grow in my heart, it would cause my heart and life to be crippled. And he said, "It is far worse to have a crippled heart and mind than a crippled body."--And I certainly agree.

I know that my family (including my grandmother, aunts and uncles), pray for me every day and I could never make it without their prayers.

As I close tonight, let me ask you to think--what brings you happiness? Maybe you have looked for it in big things instead of the smaller things in life. Perhaps you have not thought about the little things that you could do to make others happy. But, if you are seeking happiness and don't have peace, you will never find it--for peace must come first. Peace comes only from having the right relationship with our Heavenly Father and then with others.

It is my earnest prayer tonight, that each one of you will seek the right relationship with God and with others (even if you have to go to someone and apologize). Then look for and expect happiness in other things.

Fellow classmates--I wish for each of you much happiness throughout your life--but remember, happiness is not a goal--it's a by-product of other things. You'll only be as happy as you allow yourself to be."

Melany received many accolades throughout her school years. I list them here to show others what diligent hard work can accomplish even for people who are disabled and constantly in and out of the hospital. Perhaps as a mother to say how very proud we are of her because we know the great difficulties that she had in accomplishing these things.

The honors included Who's Who of American High School Students, Distinguished Society of American High School Students, National Society of High School Students, National

Honor Society, U.S. Achievement Academy, the Beta Club and the National Beta Club.

Melany also received the Georgia Tech Distinguished Science Scholar award (because she had a ninety-nine average in Science for four years). The University of Georgia Distinguished Scholar award (her overall high school average was ninety-eight).

She was on the dean's list each quarter of her college years. She was awarded the Faculty Excellence Award for the following years: 1986, 1987, 1988, 1991, 1993 and 1994. She was unable to attend college in 1989, 1990 and 1992.

She was inducted into the Bell Ringers Society and into the Honor Society PHI KAPPA PHI and was a member of the Fellowship of Christian Athletes, where she made life-time friends.

We acknowledge that she could never have achieved these things without the help of our Lord, family, friends, teachers, youth leaders and medical professionals. They helped her tremendously especially with the sustaining prayers they offered for all of us. We are very thankful and will be forever grateful.

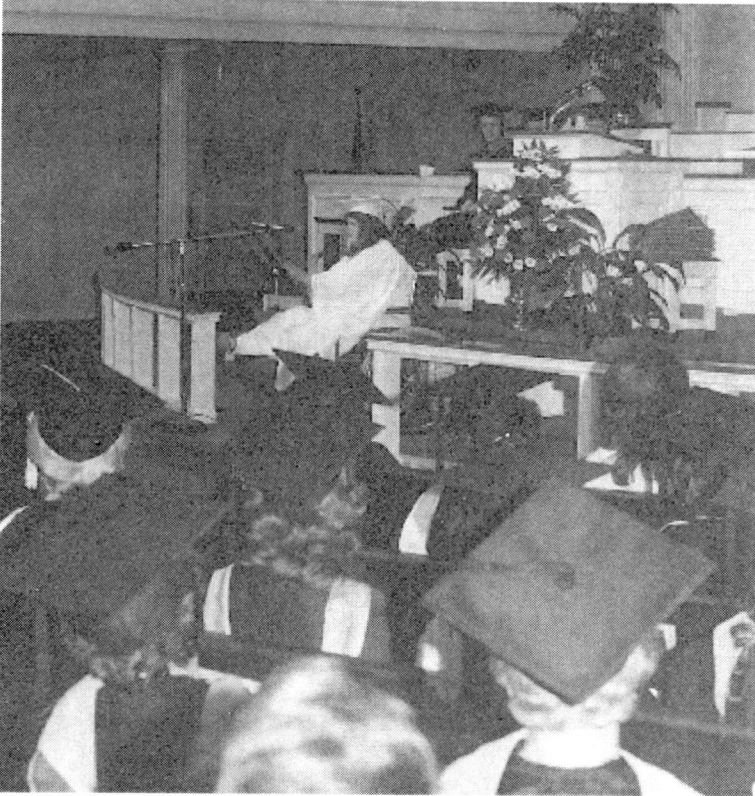

Valedictorian Address

"Joy is not in things, it is in us."
<u>*APPLES of GOLD*</u>

"The joy of the Lord is your strength."
Nehemiah 8:10b

"I can alter my life--
By altering my attitude of mind"
<u>*APPLES of GOLD*</u>

CHAPTER VI
PRAYER SUBMITTED

*"For our light affliction, which is but for a moment, worketh for
us a far more exceeding and eternal weight of glory;
While we look not at the things which are seen, but at the things
which are not seen; for the things which are seen are temporal;
but the things which are not seen are eternal."
II Corinthians 4:17 & 18.*

The summer after graduation was a wonderful time for
Melany who was full of happiness and hope, waiting until
September to go to Georgia Southern College, which is now a
University.

During the eleventh grade we had taken Missy to several
colleges to check out accessibility. She had decided in the ninth
grade she wanted to go to Georgia Southern when a representative came to visit for college day.

We went to Georgia Southern for a weekend especially
designed for eleventh graders. The ninety mile ride was on a
beautiful spring day, and the wild dogwood trees could be seen
through the many wooded areas. As we passed a fish hatchery
the road way was filled with butterflies for about a mile. I
silently thanked God that she had made it thus far.

I remember my prayer was something like this, I thanked
the Lord for sustaining her through the years. Then I prayed He
would at least allow her to get accepted to the college and be
able to attend even for a little while.

Our friends and many of our family members could not
believe we were going to allow her to go away to college and
most of them expressed their feelings to us. all of our family
members offered for her to come and stay and attend a college

near them.

We patiently explained that Augusta had a wonderful college and we would love for her to stay at home. At that time they did not have a strong program for a Therapeutic Recreation Major with a Psychology Minor.

Melany's strong desire was still to work with children in a hospital setting. She recognized that her condition was fragile and her future uncertain. She felt she could later have a small counseling office at home and help disabled children deal with hospital stays and those facing life issues living in a world with a disability.

We told everyone we felt it was more important for her to be able to pursue her dream. This would test her ability to do for herself and show us how to help her be prepared for life.

We had made many prior arrangements before school began:

FIRST, she was established with a "family," Bill and Linda Taylor. They were her parents away from home and were available and willing to help her and us with anything needed. They and their children remained Melany's friends, as long as she lived, and are very dear friends to me and Jake today.

Missy's cousins Barbara and Don Patterson lived in Statesboro with two young sons. Don was pastor of Fletcher Memorial Baptist Church that became Melany's church family away from home. All those members were good to her, and many of her FCA friends attended there.

SECOND, she had a large well equipped handicapped apartment on Sweetheart Circle in the middle of the campus.

THIRD, the college was willing to do "anything" that would help her. The administration, the professors, the maintenance staff were all so caring and giving of their time to Melany.

The administration stated they would make the campus accessible as she needed to get into different classes and areas.

FOURTH, they gave her early registration. Her dad went down as soon as she got her schedule. James, Melany, the specials needs department head and Dr. Miko her Therapeutic Recreation Advisor, toured the campus. They located her classes, and decided what was needed to get her in and out of the buildings.

Often it was just curb cuts (the campus had very few). Sometimes it involved widening doors or actually changing walls to accommodate her and her electric wheelchair. They were always so gracious and helpful.

FIFTH, we had a "caretaker" for her. Melany had a childhood friend and neighbor live with her. Melany and Mary had been friends since age two and had shared the dream of going to Southern together since the beginning of high school. Mary came from a family of four children and had attended college at home for a year. She wanted very much to go away to college.

Mary's parents paid her college fees and we paid for her housing and living expenses in exchange for her helping and caring for Melany. She would have done it for free because she had always helped her. Mary was very happy with this arrangement and so were we.

Mary shared her room with another student. Melany had a private room because she had so much adaptive "stuff." They both had private bathrooms. They had a large center living room and kitchen which became the center of many gatherings and many lasting friendships were made.

Mary had a big responsibility in caring for Melany and always did a fantastic job! Mary will probably never realize this side of Heaven what a blessing she was to Melany and to us. Without her help Melany could not have started to college there nor continued later.

It was a wonderful day when both families moved the girls to Statesboro. It was a dream come true and an answer to many prayers. We were all excited and very thankful!

Within days they were happily settled and anticipating great times. Melany had an electric wheelchair and a new van she could drive with hand controls. She always had a group of friends with her and they called it "the happy bus."

We called her electric wheelchair "the tank" or "the all-terrain vehicle." She could go through fields and wooded areas in it however she occasionally met difficulties.

Several changes were made to the campus buildings. One of her classes was in a portable class room and a ramp was built at the back door. The walking students used the front door but Melany had to drive her chair to the back and cross a large grassy area.

There were heavy rains during one weekend, when class started on Monday they missed Melany. She was found sitting in the wheelchair in the pouring rain stuck in the middle of the grassy area.

Some of the large football players went and lifted her and the heavy wheelchair into the classroom.

Missy was soaking wet but they said she just laughed and said, "God always sends me angels when I need them. But they are not usually this good looking."

Another very frightening incident happened one Friday afternoon during a late class. Mary had come home for the weekend to attend a wedding. Most of her close friends had either gone home for the weekend or to a concert in Savannah. Melany had stayed at school by herself feeling very independent. She had a late class and needed to finish a class project. She also had an "important" date on Saturday Night. The class was having a movie on the second floor of the library where she had never been. Her classmates all went up the stairs. There was no regular elevator so the receptionist took Melany up in the back service elevator. Melany did not realize the elevator had a keyed switch to enter and to run it.

After the movie the instructor and class members went down the stairs. Melany went down the narrow hall to the elevator but there was no button to push. She realized she was alone on the second floor of a soundproof building. The viewing room was on the back side of the building overlooking a small lake and a wooded area and no one would be able to see or hear her. The doors to the rooms on the front of the building were locked.

Melany said she just tried to remain calm and started asking God to help her. She went back into the viewing room where a student had returned to retrieve the notebook he had left there. She said she was so glad to see him she practically attacked him, fearful that he would run out again.

He (like so many other helpers) assured her he would get the people down stairs to bring the elevator for her. The young man came back and stayed with her until security came. This experience taught her to watch out for keyed elevators.

Melany had endeared herself to many students and faculty members with her humble attitude and delightful sense of humor. This continued through her nine years of college life. Her dad always laughingly said he thought she was going to be a perpetual student.

Many prayers sustained her and her first quarter of college was delightful but also very physically difficult. She pushed herself and her fragile muscles beyond endurance. When she came home for the Christmas Holidays she went directly into the hospital where she stayed for many months.

It was hard to believe her life had touched so many people on a college campus in only one quarter. Cards and letters of encouragement came every day. Every weekend several of her friends and other students some who had only met her briefly, drove the hour and a half trip to the hospital to visit her.

Melany was active in the Fellowship of Christian Athletes. One of the officers of FCA said that practically every dormitory on campus was meeting in their basement recreation rooms having a prayer meeting for Melany every night!

She said people who were not even Christians were joining and praying for her healing and for her to be able to return to campus.

As the groups voluntarily formed they began praying for themselves, each other, their families and school needs.

Some of the dorm groups had asked for members from FCA to come and help them get started, because they did not know how to pray.

A prayer revival was breaking out on campus! The local and school newspapers had articles about it.

From the last week of November through the first week in February Melany had three vascular strokes.

Her body was so grotesquely drawn that her arms were drawn up to her chest and she could only move one hand. One of her legs was drawn completely up. Later the other one drew also, like she was sitting "Indian Style" with her legs crossed.

Her head was drawn back and her eyes drawn upward looking toward the left. We had to stand at the head of her bed for her to see us.

The worst part was she was unable to speak for a long time. It was hard not knowing if she was in more pain (she was always in pain) or if she was hot, cold or thirsty.

Melany's Occupational Therapist, Emily, and her Speech Therapist, Jan, made her a spelling board. These are often used in hospitals now.

When we held the board under her hand that she could use, and up for her to be able to see it, she could point to symbols or letters. It was a slow process when she tried to spell a word but with patience it worked. On one side were the letters of the alphabet and on the other side were symbols such as doctor, nurse, pain, potty, hot, cold, thirsty, food, mom, family, friend, preacher, and a few others. This was very helpful.

A very dear doctor had her to slowly blink once for "yes," twice for "no," and rapidly for "I don't know or please repeat." This was also a big help.

When the otolaryngologist examined her she had no gag reflex when he put his instrument all the way to her vocal chords. He said her muscles had let go and her vocal chords were "floppy" and could not be fixed.

Melany's muscles would spasm constantly. Every spasm was a very painful visible ripple that often went from her neck down her body to her toes.

When she could still speak she had expressed that every spasm felt like a "charley horse" we experience in the calves of our legs. Her mouth would open sideways but no audible scream came out and big tears would roll down her cheeks.

The physical therapist said the trapezius muscle was involved. This is a large muscle that would normally spasm, hold for a few seconds or a minute then relax and let go. The Behcet's involvement interfered with the brain sensors and was not sending the signal to relax.

The attending doctors tried every known medication for spasms and pain but nothing worked. The spasms and pain were relentless day and night.

For her nineteenth birthday all Melany wanted was a few hours of relief from pain but it was one of her worst days.

The doctors had called a meeting with her primary doctor, Dr. Magruder, surgeon, Dr. Engler, gastroenterologist, Dr. Pitts, orthopedist, Dr. Goodwin, and neurologist, Dr. McClure, all who were working together trying to help her.

The plans were for an anesthesiologist to put her to sleep and the neurologist and orthopedic surgeon would insert a catheter into her spine with an opening and a port left outside the spine. They would keep it filled with medication to numb her pain. It would have to be refilled several times a day. Several years later some other doctors perfected a similar procedure with the drug Baclofen. At that time they had nothing to offer except the epidural-like treatment.

They had spoken with the anesthesiologist the day before and they were gathering to discuss with him the pros and cons of this unorthodox procedure.

James and I had already signed several legal papers stating they could try anything to help ease her. We felt we had no choice as she had not slept more than a few minutes at a time for several days and nights.

The anesthesiologist was a very delightful and interesting person who was also caring and inquisitive. One of the doctors had spoken with him the evening before and he read everything he could find about Behcet's. His wife told me later he had read most of the night. He had never heard of the disease before so he was interested in it.

He came to the meeting with grim news. He had learned that because of the vast and delicate involvement of all the nerve cells and nerve endings they could not administer the numbing medicine. It was almost certain that her entire central nervous system would shut down and she would be unable to move and would possibly be left in an irreversible vegetative or comatose state.

All her doctors were very distressed but they were grateful he had found that information before they tried the procedure.

We thanked the Lord for making us aware of these possibilities. James and I expressed that to the disappointed doctors and thanked them for trying.

As we walked into the hall, her orthopedic doctor who had cared for her since she was twelve years old just broke down and cried. He said, "I cannot believe that I am standing in one of the best medical facilities with every muscle or pain reliever known to man available and I can find nothing to ease this child."

I said to James, "When your doctor cries, you know you are in real trouble." We looked at each other and smiled because we have always tried to keep a sense of humor especially in very difficult circumstances.

As we again submitted Melany to the Lord we prayed He would make a better way to help her. We knew she had submitted her life to God and her trust was in Him.

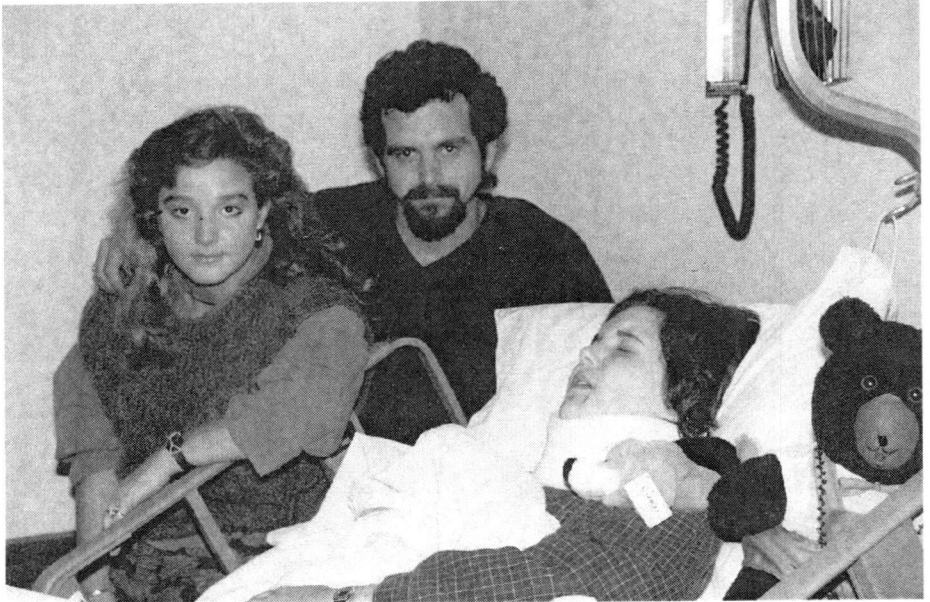

Kim and Ric with Melany

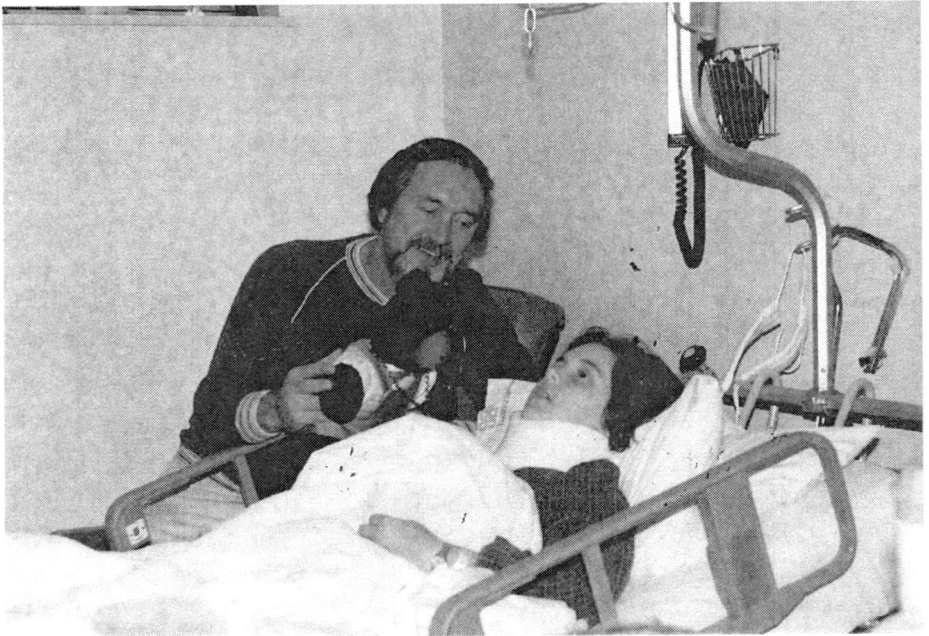

Dad and Melany

The anesthesiologist, Dr. Joe Garrison came in around six

o'clock that evening and said "I believe I can ease this child, even temporarily." He explained he was using a drug in the operating room to relieve extensive muscle spasms. It was used in hip or other joint replacements and for some spinal surgery and relieved severe short-term spasms. The name of the medication was Buprenex. It had only been approved by the FDA since the second of January to be used in our state outside of the operating room and this was the thirtieth of January. How good God is!

Dr. Garrison had spoken with the other doctors who said he could try it if we agreed. We asked Melany if she wanted to try it. She said she did. We prayed about it and agreed to do it. Our lawyer, Lou Saul, came immediately and drew up many papers relieving the hospital, drug company, doctors, and everyone from any liability.

Dr. Garrison sat by her bed and very, very slowly injected the medication into her IV line. He started about eight o'clock and finished after two a.m.

He would slowly inject the medication, pause for about five minutes and start again. It was truly like watching a miracle.

Her body began slowly relaxing and her arms came down, her leg relaxed and she could turn her head slightly. We were all exuberant. Missy slept for twelve hours as she was completely exhausted and sleep deprived.

The nurses continued administering the medicine every two hours to keep her body relaxed. They did have to splint her leg and arms to keep them straight because the muscles had been tight for so long.

Even though her birthday had been one of the most pain filled days she had ever endured, the day after was wonderful by comparison. She still had a lot of pain but the muscles were relaxing and it was bearable.

All of us, especially Melany and the doctors were ecstatic. However, Dr. Garrison reminded us they had not used this for long-term muscle relaxing and they were not sure how long it could be used. They didn't even know for sure how it would affect her cognitive abilities.

Dr. Garrison's theory was, the problem was not what they could see that was wrong, it was what they couldn't see. He explained that the Pseudocholinesrerase that balanced the muscles was imbalanced. He said that he had seen this as he worked with spinal cord injuries and with polio victims years ago. The example he gave was, "when my leg gets a muscle spasm, something tells it to let go after a while." Melany's doesn't say "let go," it is not working right. He said that the Morphine receptors in her brain had been destroyed either from the episodes she had suffered, or from the Behcet's Disease. He said that the Buprenex fills up the morphine receptors, when they are full, the excess is eliminated.

We were all thankful for every day, even every hour and minute that her muscles were relaxed.

Since she had the three vascular strokes she had difficulty swallowing. The paralysis from her vocal chords seemed to be moving down into her esophagus. Within a week after her birthday the doctors said that they were getting concerned about her swallowing and felt we needed to send her to a major diagnostic center. They made the necessary arrangements and told us we were to leave by air ambulance the next morning at 6:30 a.m.

Our family and friends have often teased us (especially my husband) about us being so frugal. How thankful I was that we were careful with our spending and that my husband could write a check for the $7,000.00 (a lot of money in 1985) ambulance fee that night. Of course, this was for one way. But I knew he would get us back.

Once again James had to stay home and work so we could afford the needed care. James was very uneasy about Melany and me going alone. We had always been very close and I could almost read his mind. Finally I said to him, "I know the feelings and fears you have about Melany. But I know also that you are concerned about me. You know that if Melany dies, I will be all alone thousands of miles from home. If something should happen to her, just remember what we have always known and had proven to us time and again, 'God's grace is always sufficient.' He will be with me and I will be alright.

I do not want you to try to come to me. If you cannot send a plane for me, I will get a commercial flight and come home. I will be OK."

Choose by faith, To create a new life
within this Unexpected frame work."
FINDING HOPE WHEN LIFE'S NOT FAIR

Is there not something captivating in the sight of a man or woman burdened with many tribulations and yet carrying a heart as sound as a bell?
Is there not something contagiously valorous in the vision of one who is greatly tempted, but is more than conqueror?
Is it not heartening to see some pilgrim who is broken in body, but who retains the splendor of an unbroken patience?
What a witness all this offers to the endurement of His grace!
J. H. Jowett
STREAMS IN THE DESERT

CHAPTER VII
PRAYER SUBLIME

"Do as Thou hast said--That thy name may be magnified
for ever.--I Chronicles 17:23b & 24a

"He answered no thing." Mark 15:3

The next morning when we arrived at the airport we had
quite a send off. James and Ric were there, along with Melany's
Physical Therapist, Sally, her Occupational Therapist, Emily, her
Speech Therapist, Jan, and one of her doctors. Our friends Joyce
and Roy and Missy's friends Joey and Mike were there also.
They all cried as we left. I did not cry until we were in the air
and I was sure Melany was alright. The flight was miserable.
The "air ambulance" was simply a small two prop plane which
normally carried six passengers. They had removed one side of
the seats for a stretcher. It was very cold and the nurse and I
wore heavy jackets, hoods and gloves.

I had never flown in a small plane before and as day light
came I was amazed to be able to see the ground, houses and cars.
I thought something must be wrong with the plane for us to be
flying so low. I asked the nurse about it. She did not know
because she had never flown before either. I just went back to
sleep. I reasoned that if we were going to crash, I couldn't do
anything about it and if I was asleep then I wouldn't know it. I
have always been teased about my ability to sleep anytime,
anywhere.

When I awoke again and realized we had not crashed, I
really enjoyed the view. The country- side view from the air was
lovely with the snow covering everything. We landed in
Champaign, Illinois, for refueling and a snack.

We arrived in Rochester, Minnesota around 4:30 p.m. It was

bitterly cold so they pulled the plane into the hangar and loaded us into the waiting ambulance.

The evening we arrived the doctor ordered pain medicine and muscle relaxants for Melany. He said they would not be using the Buprenex but other medicines. They had some special therapy they wanted to try.

It was 12:30 a.m. when the tired, over-worked yet very dedicated young resident came in to take her history. His last name was Merritt (my maiden name) and he had gone to medical school in Augusta and visited the singles Sunday School Class that I had taught. I have often wondered what happened to that fine young doctor.

Melany was very ill and I was so very tired. I had only eaten a package of crackers all day. There was no cafeteria or snack bar at St. Mary's, and the snack machines were far away and I was too tired to go. A sweet nurse's aide had brought me some crackers and a coke about ten o'clock and I was very grateful.

The same aide's church members supplied meals for people like me that were stranded at the hospital. They brought a dinner meal every night except Saturday and Sunday. They were so sweet and kind and I was so appreciative.

I was also thankful to be in one of the finest hospitals in the world with Melany. It was quite obvious it was one of the best because there were many people including a lot of doctor's family members from around the world being diagnosed and treated.

Melany's room was across from the neuro-intensive care waiting room. The vistors would gather there three times a day for the visiting times.

When the staff was working with Melany I would go over and visit with some of the visitors, especially those that were alone or lonely. I heard many wonderful reports of miracles happening there through the fine physicians. Of course there were many heartaches, disappointments and deaths.

I thanked and praised the Lord because I just knew they

were going to be able to help my dear daughter.

The next few days many doctors and therapists did many tests and tried several things. They even had a machine with electric paddles that was supposed to release the spasms.

Missy's one leg kept drawing tighter and tighter in the heavy brace that was relentlessly holding it.

All the doctors, nurses and therapists were good and very compassionate except this one doctor that was over this particular part of her care.

When nothing was working to relieve the spasms and pain, I finally spoke up and asked why they were not using the Buprenex, because we knew that it worked to relieve the spasms.

All of the medicines except one they were using had already been tried and was documented in the records that we had brought from Georgia.

The head doctor was very abrupt with me and told me in no uncertain tones they would not be using Buprenex at all, and to please not mention this to them again.

In all the years Melany had been sick and during the many hospitalizations, we had never had a disagreement with a doctor. We had one that seemed to have a bad attitude occasionally but we knew he was an excellent physician and cared for his patients.

This doctor was different and was rude and arrogant with us, the staff and even his contemporaries. It was obvious he had not studied the thick pack of records our doctors and hospital had so carefully prepared and sent with us. He referred to our good dedicated doctors as the "Good old Georgia Boys." This did not set well with me at all. All of our doctors were dedicated, very efficient and professional. Although I tried, my attitude with him was not the best and I apologized to him later.

The doctor said the doctors in Augusta had contributed to her vascular condition by allowing me to take her from doctor to doctor and get various pain medications often for days in a row.

He also said that as a mother I was giving in to her because she was still taking children's chewable vitamins. I was completely baffled by this diagnosis and tried in vain to speak with him.

The doctor had the leg brace removed and tried the paddle machine again. Her knee was cut with deep gashes and was bleeding where it had drawn repeatedly against the unyielding support. It would not straighten and only drew up more so the heel was actually tight against her private area. That made it almost impossible to get her on a bedpan. The doctor was very upset and said they WOULD get it straightened.

I told the young doctor that to get it straightened in Augusta they had to put her to sleep. I had told him when he took her information and it was in the records that I had brought. He said the head doctor said that was not necessary and he had to follow his instructions. I also told him that the leg would never stay straight without the Buprenex. He told me the main doctor did not want to tell me but Buprenex was only approved in that state to be used in the operating room and in the intensive care unit. That explanation would have certainly helped me to understand about the medication if the head doctor had only told me. I would not have angered him by asking again.

They cleaned her leg and the young doctor and two nurses gave her valium intravenously and tried to straighten the leg. They asked me to leave. They worked for about thirty minutes and all came out sweating profusely and both nurses were crying.

The doctor said, "Never again!" One of the nurses said that it was almost more than they could endure. They knew the pain was excruciating and when Melany opened her mouth to scream nothing came out. They could not make the leg move at all.

When I went into Melany's room to comfort her she was completely exhausted and looked like the victims of torture that you see on television. She was in so much pain she was almost delirious

I had never felt so sad, alone and defeated in my life. I was having long talks with the Lord.

All of the other doctors were superb. As I spoke with them they were all understanding and very kind, but they could not go over the head doctor. Melany was getting weaker and she could hardly swallow and was begging to go home.

Finally one of the older doctors told me, "If she was my daughter, I would take her back to her doctors in Georgia where you know that you can get medication that helped."

We were there for Valentine's. James and Ric sent us a big arrangement of red roses and very sweet cards. James called and told us both how very special we were and how much he loved us every day not just on Valentine's Day. That helped my feelings a lot but Melany was to weak and sick to respond to much.

Many of our friends sent flowers, gifts and cards. Dr. Sautel and Dr. McFagen, two of our favorite doctors brought her a bear and an angel. Dr. Sautel's wife had made her a heart-shaped cake, but she was unable to eat any of it. The staff and I enjoyed it very much.

Melany was getting weaker and weaker. After lunch I was reading through my spiral notebook that I wrote in every day. I had a copy of her valedictorian address folded in the book. I read it to her and asked if she still believed what she had written about faith, peace, happiness and joy. She blinked her eyes indicating that she did and asked for "the board" where she spelled ABSOLUTELY. I reminded her of the many people who said they were blessed by it. I said, "Missy you can't be robbed of your peace and joy now. Remember you said the joy of the Lord is deep inside of us and it will surface again." She blinked yes and I said, "Please my darling hold on to that."

I read Psalm 121 (one of her favorites) to her. One of the doctors came and motioned for me to come out into the hall. He took me into the empty waiting room where four other doctors and two of the therapists were waiting.

The doctor in charge said they had believed they could help

her but there was nothing more they could do at this time. Every Valentine's Day I re-read what I wrote in my devotional book that night. The doctor had said, "You cannot manage her care at home. It takes four nurses and aides to put her on the bedpan and six to turn her and to change her bed." He continued, "Just take her back to the hospital in Augusta and see if they can help ease her pain. If she lives more than a couple of months then put her in a nursing home until the end. It will not be long because her body is shutting down."

He said they had a few other things they could try if I wanted them to but they were not really sure they would help. Once again they each expressed their regrets and a couple patted me and two of them hugged me just as the doctors had done ten years before at Johns Hopkins. They left me alone and this time they did not even send the chaplain in. I wept bitterly!

I have always had too much love and respect coupled with a healthy amount of fear to lash out at God but I was so hurt and afraid. In counseling I have often told people, "God understands our pain and our bad attitudes and He still wants to help us if we allow Him to."

I said in essence, "God, how could you let this happen? I think you have really blown it. Lord, just one little miracle from you. I did not even ask for complete healing. Just that she live and be restored back to where she was, and be able to return to school.

Don't you know, Lord, that we have been told that there are college students who never pray and don't even know you, yet they are gathering praying for Melany. Just think God, (I'm telling God to think) many could be brought to you with just one little miracle from you."

I truly felt that the Heavens were as brass. I had left my devotional book in the waiting room earlier that day and when I picked it up I "happened" to turn to the Scripture *"I called Him, but he gave me no answer."* Song of Solomon 5:6. Then I flipped the pages and read.

The writer H. Bonar said, *"The Lord, when He hath given great faith, hath been known to try it by long delayings. He has suffered His servants' voices to echo in their ears as from a brazen sky. They have knocked at the golden gate, but it has remained unmovable, as though it were rusted upon its hinges. Like Jeremiah, they have cried, 'Thou has covered thyself with a cloud, that our prayer should not pass through.' Thus have true saints continued long in patient waiting without reply, not because their prayers were not vehement, nor because they were unaccepted, but because it so pleased Him who is Sovereign, and who gives according to His own pleasure. If it pleases Him to bid our patience exercise itself, shall He not do as He will with His own!*

No prayer is lost. Praying breath was never spent in vain. There is no such thing as prayer unanswered or unnoticed by God, and some things that we count refusals or denials are simply delays."

I said, "Oh God, I am so sorry, so very sorry for the way I talked to you. I'm just so scared and I'm two thousand miles from home (I'm still telling God facts) and people that really care about us and I'm so disappointed and hurt. Please forgive me."

I started across to Melany's room and they were still working with her. I stood looking out of the large plate glass window at the end of the hall. I thought about teaching singles and singles again back home. I always tell them when things are really bad to look to God and find one good thing to focus on and give God thanks and praise Him for it. Continue doing that until your faith returns.

Out the window in the beautiful falling snow I saw boys and girls and happy families sledding down this lovely sloping hill. I thanked God and praised Him for the happy children. I looked at each one of them and asked Him to bless them and keep them healthy and to bless their parents and protect them from the pain I was feeling because of the pain my child was experiencing.

I thanked God for all the beauty I saw in the snow covered trees, which looked like a winter wonderland.

When I went back into the waiting room to get a tissue they were hanging a large picture over the sofa. It was printed to look like cross stitch and it simply said,

*"It's because of the things that
I can see and understand,
That I can trust Him with the
Things I cannot see and understand."*

I went back into Melany's room with a renewed faith. She was lying very still but I could see her move her one finger in a sort of triangular motion. I watched as she was signing the hymn over and over with her finger, *"It will be worth it all, when we see Jesus."*

I went down the hall to the pay phone and called our Dr. Magruder in Augusta. I told him that Melany was getting worse and they were not helping her. I told him what the other doctor had suggested about bringing her back to Georgia. He was always so sweet and kind. He said, "I agree, just bring her on back home and we will do our best to help her." What a comfort he was!

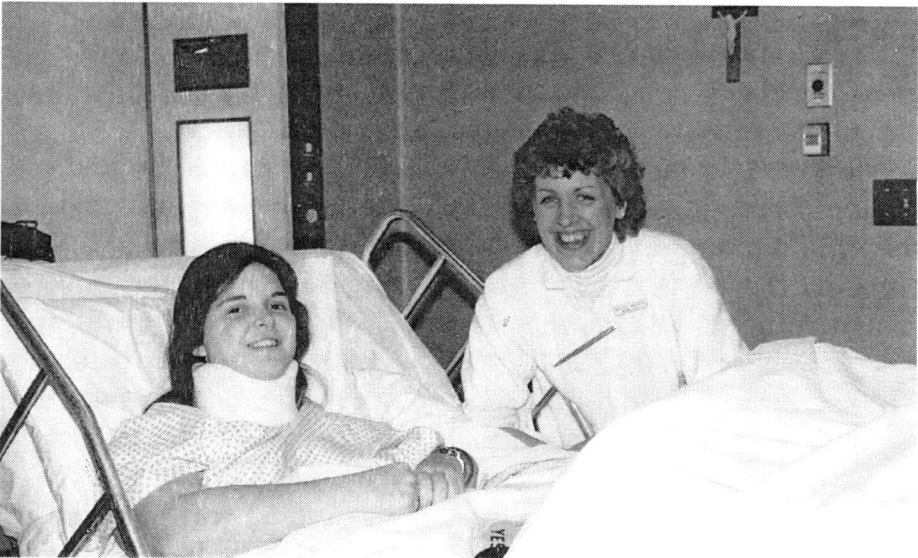

Melany with a nurse at Mayo

Nancy Wiggins

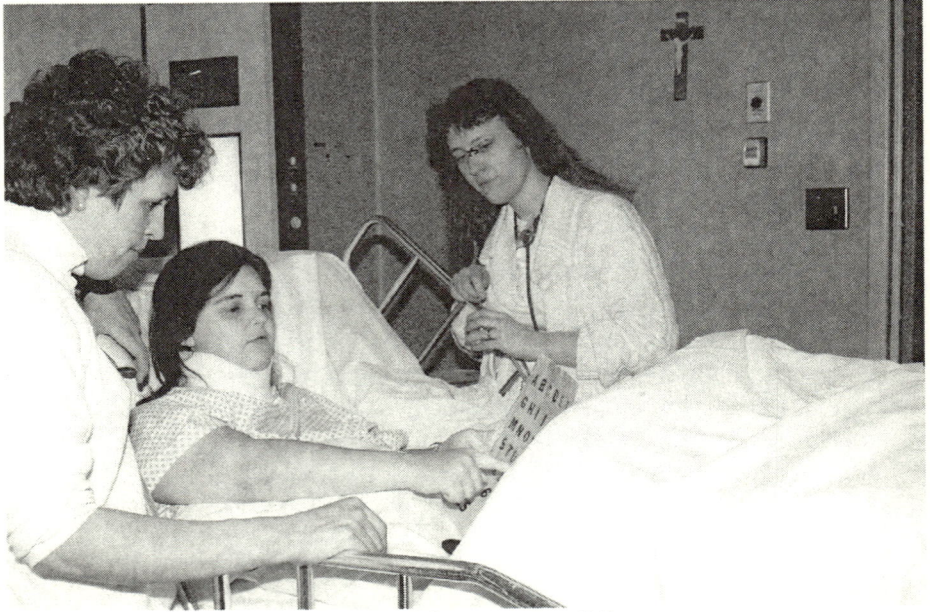

Melany with nurses at Mayo

I called James and it was like *deja vu* from John Hopkins. We cried together when I had to tell him that nothing could be done and to please make arrangements to come and get us.

I never told James how badly I felt I was treated by that one doctor. I just prayed and asked God to forgive him and tried to forget it. I thought I had until I started writing this book. When I got to the notes I had made during that time, the pain of remembrance was almost unbearable and I prayed through it again. Perhaps the incident somehow made me a better person.

The next day we didn't see any doctors. I learned later one of the doctors had talked to the head doctor and asked him to take a closer look at Melany's records that day.

On Sunday the head doctor came in and he was much nicer. He said he had studied her records more closely, and he would like to talk to me about some things. He also seemed ready to listen to me and I was able to share the following with him:

1. She only started taking chewable children's vitamins after the strokes because she could not swallow the others.

2. She had been in the hospital for three and a half months. All the pain medicines and muscle relaxants had been given by her own doctors plus different doctors who were on call when the nurses would call them because the previous medications were not working. I wanted him to understand I had not initiated any of this.

The doctor did give me a half-hearted apology and admitted that he had "missed some parts of the transcript." He said he really had thought they could help her and was very sorry they could not.

I apologized for my bad attitude and told him how confused I was by his statements because we had used the same doctors for years and I had always left the medications up to them. I also told him that we had some of the finest doctors in Augusta, and I felt he was out of line in talking about them and questioning their decisions. He said perhaps he was not as well informed as he should have been.

I told Melany that her daddy was coming to get us. She was so happy and she tried to smile but only one corner of her mouth would go up, almost looking like a snarl.

James rented a much nicer plane and he and Ric came to get us. I had never been so glad to see him in all of our days together, as I was that day. The head doctor talked to them and he was very nice to us.

Thus, we left one of the top and finest medical centers in the world very disappointed, but still trusting God. We were very grateful that Melany was still with us.

The dictionary describes sublime as:

1. Exalted, noble.

2. Having awe-inspiring beauty or grandeur

Once again our friends, family, church family, neighbors and students at Melany's college had offered high and exalted and noble prayers to our Heavenly Father. The prayers indeed had awe-inspiring beauty and grandeur that we did not realize fully for a long time.

We acknowledged that prayer sublime does not always bring the miracles or answers that we seek, or desire, but it does bring peace to our hearts and minds!

> *"Disappointment with God is a process*
> *in which the soul can be torn apart*
> *and patched together again."*
> **FINDING HOPE WHEN LIFE IS NOT FAIR**

> *"A loving Father whispers,*
> *'This cometh from my hand,'*
> *Blessed are ye if ye trust*
> *Where you cannot understand."*
> **STREAMS IN THE DESERT**

CHAPTER VIII
<u>PRAISE</u>

"Let us offer the sacrifice of praise
to   God continually. Hebrews 13:15

We returned home to our wonderful caring doctors. Melany stayed in the hospital for three additional months using the Buprenex which relaxed her muscles and helped with the pain. A feeding tube was implanted into her stomach to infuse nourishment as she still could not swallow very well. A type of port-a-cath called a "Groshong" catheter was inserted into her chest. With the catheter the muscle relaxing medicine was released continually through a Cad Pump. The medication was evenly distributed which prevented having a shot every three or four hours.

I cannot say I have always been able to praise and thank God *for* my circumstances and difficulties. I have always been able to be thankful and praise Him *in* my circumstances and difficulties.

Sometimes in our pain and heartaches praise is a sacrifice. We can offer this sacrifice of praise unto the Lord because God is always worthy of our praise.

Many prayers are answered through our praise and we are told in Psalm 22:3, *"The Lord inhabits the praise of His people."*

We began really concentrating on praising the Lord in worship and prayer. Every day we looked for and found something to focus on to praise God for. Such as creation, our salvation, sustaining grace, our family, friends, caring doctors, nurses and staff, Buprenex, the Groshong Catheter, the feeding tube, our church family and staff, freedoms we have and enjoy in our country, and popsicles (Melany ate a lot of those). We could offer sincere praise and thanksgiving especially for every small improvement in her condition.

One of our greatest continual praises came when she was able to speak again. All our friends, family and doctors rejoiced!

Melany was finally able to go home which was another great praise. During the summer many of her friends from college visited her as well as those at home. She was still very weak and they offered much encouragement to her.

We went to St. Simons Island, her favorite place for several weeks. We had never been for an extended stay during the summer because we always rented our condo as often as possible to help make the monthly payments. Her dad felt she certainly deserved this trip. On the fourth of July we could sit on the beach and view fireworks in four directions, what fun we all had.

Several of her friends from home and school came to visit for a few days. Melany enjoyed every minute of the stay.

We continued praising God and thanking Him. Melany did return to school in the fall with much praising and rejoicing again!

Melany's doctors agreed for her to go to school if I went and stayed until I was sure she and Mary could handle the situation. Those two girls could handle any situation and had done so since before they were in playschool.

We had the usual Wiggins-Faulk "preschool-instructional" meeting with Melany and Mary, which I'm sure the girls followed explicitly. We had laughingly remembered how determined they were as little girls. One of our neighbors across the creek had a horse. The girls went almost every day and fed the horse through the fence. We had an unusually cold icy winter. Our seven and eight year olds did not feel the horse had proper shelter. Without discussing it with us, they called the animal control services and reported it. They had called from our phone and given our address. Of course the officers came to my door to fill out a report that I knew nothing of. Melany and Mary were there, so they filled in all the details. I was very embarrassed because they went to the neighbors and threatened to remove the horse if proper measures were not taken. I reprimanded the girls and assured them that if they had talked this over with an adult, we would have talked to the neighbors. I reminded them that the neighbors were very caring people who cared for several animals and they would have corrected the situation. They told me not to worry, they had handled it, and they continued to check on the horse daily. This was the same neighbor that owned the cat that Melany had painted when she was younger. We maintained a good relationship through the years, I'm not sure how!

Then we recalled that when they were in middle school (Melany's first year), and Melany was using crutches and a scooter, her knee cap kept coming out of place. We took her to the Orthopedic Doctor a couple of times, and Mary went with us (they went everywhere together). After observing, they decided that they could get it in place themselves. They did a good job, which was a blessing because sometimes it happened daily. The doctor was apprehensive at first. But after x-raying the knee admitted that they had been successful in not "nicking" or "chipping" the knee cap. He was very surprised, as he said it was difficult for professionals to avoid this sometimes. Later, after several surgeries this was corrected, then she went into the wheelchair full time, so it was not a problem. We knew for certain that those two could handle "anything" and most situations.

Once again, the Wiggins-Faulk caravan headed for Statesboro. It consisted of James and F.M. (Mary's dad) driving their overloaded trucks, Mildred (Mary's mom) and me in my car, Mary and her brother David in her car and Ric driving Melany in her van. What a happy group we were!

Mildred and I were praising and thanking the Lord that our girls were returning to school. We were thankful Mildred was able to go as she had a heart transplant the year before and could not travel last fall.

When Melany was so ill in January we had asked our deacons to come lay hands on her and pray for healing. I told Mildred I had shared a letter two weeks ago with Melany reminding her of the invitation James and I had sent to our deacons in our church and some elders in a couple of other churches including Melany's church in Statesboro.

Our request read as follows:

PLEASE COME TO ST. JOSEPH HOSPITAL ON SUNDAY JANUARY 18, 1986, at 2:00 p.m. TO LAY HANDS ON MELANY AND PRAY FOR:

(1) Ease of severe spasms and pain. (Buprenex did that on January 31.)

(2) Her voice to be restored. (She regained her ability to speak in April.)

(3) Be able to straighten her fingers and use her hands again. (The use was slowly returning.)

(4) That her vision would clear and she could focus her eyes again. (That had happened gradually.)

(5) Her desire to return to college. (That was happening now!)

At the requested time the deacons had gathered in the lobby of the hospital and prayed. Then led by the hospital Chaplain Father Muns, our pastor Rev. John Bryan, and chairman of our deacons Roy Scarborough they went in pairs down the hall to Melany's room. What an impression these Godly men made on the entire floor as they were obedient to the scripture.

The doctors, nurses, staff members and visitors stood in awe and silence as the men proceeded to Melany's room prayed for her and returned to the lobby and knelt in prayer until all thirty of them had finished. God is faithful and He does answer our prayers in His own time and His own way. Some of those who witnessed that scene still share with us years later what a spiritual blessing it was to them.

I had written a note to all the men the next week thanking them and sharing the marvelous way that God had answered their prayers. Mildred and I continued praising and thanking God.

While unloading all the vehicles the dads repeated what

they said last fall they had never seen two girls with so many clothes and shoes. They helped Mary and me get the boxes into the various rooms. We all went to our favorite seafood restaurant before the tired crew left.

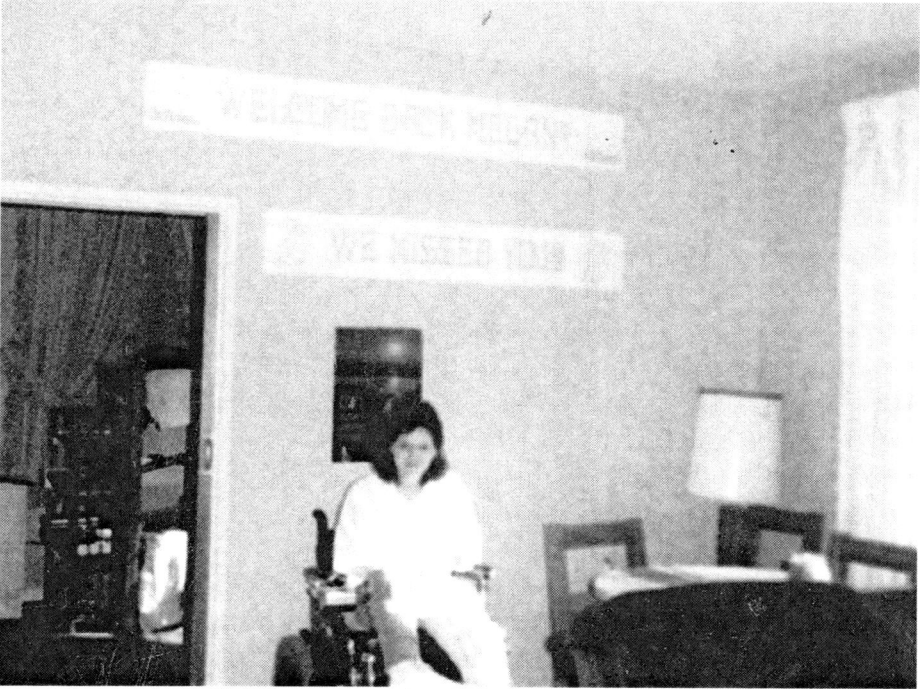

Welcome back Melany, we missed you - a welcome back to college

I stayed for two more weeks. Melany did need a little extra help with bathing, her leg and arm supports, the feedings, cleaning the feeding tube, Groshong Catheter, etc.

Mary had extra things to deal with but the chest catheter would free her of having to coordinate her schedule with Melany's for her shots every three to four hours. Also she would not have to get up during the night. We knew that Melany would soon be able to take responsibility for cleaning her catheter and her feeding tube and even do her own feedings. She still could eat some food and could also suction herself.

During the few times she had to suction herself in her

classrooms half of the students had to leave. Dr. Miko chided them explaining to them that as health professionals they were likely to be confronted with patients being suctioned and perhaps would have to assist with the procedure. I'm sure they did not want to hear that as it was not a very pleasant thing to do.

Melany and Mary had gone to school early and had several days to get settled and visit with everyone. They had their schedules but they were most interested in getting their social life organized.

The first day we had been very busy getting the apartment organized. The next morning Melany in her electric wheelchair and I on very tired feet took a stroll around the campus. She was anxious to see who was already there and to visit with her friends. We had to check out her classes and determine what was needed.

Melany had a soft neck brace to help support her head. Her legs were extended with braces securing them to be sure they did not draw up because of her additional moving around. Both arms had supports also. She looked a wreck but she was at college and everyone was happy for her!

One of her dear Christian friends met us on the sidewalk. She had a precious young classmate with her that did not know Melany.

In her excited little voice, Margie said "Oh, Melany, we have prayed so long and hard for you. Isn't it wonderful that God has restored you, healed you and brought you back to school?"

The other girl looked at Melany with very wide eyes and said in her adorable dialect "Youse healed?" I guess she thought, 'If Melany is healed don't pray for me!'

Melany's second day was so exciting and the apartment was filled with well wishers all day and half of the night. Those young people never sleep!

I had met with the special needs director and he arranged for four recliners we had purchased to be placed in her classrooms. These were necessary for although her spasms were relieved she still had severe pain in her back and could not sit in the wheelchair for very long. The director had also had the carpenters in the shop make sliding boards to leave with each recliner so Melany could transfer from her wheelchair without having to carry a board around. What thoughtfulness all the staff extended.

The first day of classes Melany was eager to start as she wanted to see her teachers and classmates. One of her classes was on Death and Dying. She had heard a lot about her professor who was quite flamboyant in his style of teaching and his methods were also very direct.

He began the class by stating how wrong he felt it was to keep people "alive" with extreme measures. He expressed the quality of life was much more important for patients, their families, society, and taxpayers than the quantity was.

He went on to say that today they had people depending on breathing with oxygen who were barely alive. In the hospitals they poke tubes in every hole a person has and make some additional holes just to put tubes in. Everyone laughed.

He looked over in the corner of the room and spied Melany. There she sat in her recliner by her wheelchair. She had all her braces, tubes, oxygen and suction machine on and around her. The other students said he was so embarrassed he was speechless, a new experience for him I am sure. Melany just smiled sweetly at him and gave him the "back to you" sign. They became great friends and taught each other many things that quarter and their friendship continued until her graduation.

When I was sure Melany and Mary could take care of everything, I was very ready to go home. My college experience had been tiring, lots of fun, and very interesting and enlightening. I slept on one of the couches in their living room. It was always late when I went to sleep because people were there until half of the night. One morning I awoke and saw a strange young man on the couch opposite mine. I grabbed my robe and quickly slipped into Melany's room and woke her with the news. She was not surprised and said, "Oh, it is probably Kirby. Last year he came and slept here when his roommate had overnight company so we always leave our door unlocked in case anyone needs to sleep in the living room." I was surprised that they could have people stay overnight in Kirby's and other apartments. I was horrified that these three "intelligent" girls were so careless. I decided I needed to leave before I learned any more.

In the fall Statesboro had a city wide revival sponsored by several churches. They had a wonderful night for the youth and college students. They provided music that appealed to them. Those in charge of the planning had asked Melany to be one of the speakers and share some of the things that God's grace had given her. She was introduced by our dear friend, Bill Taylor.

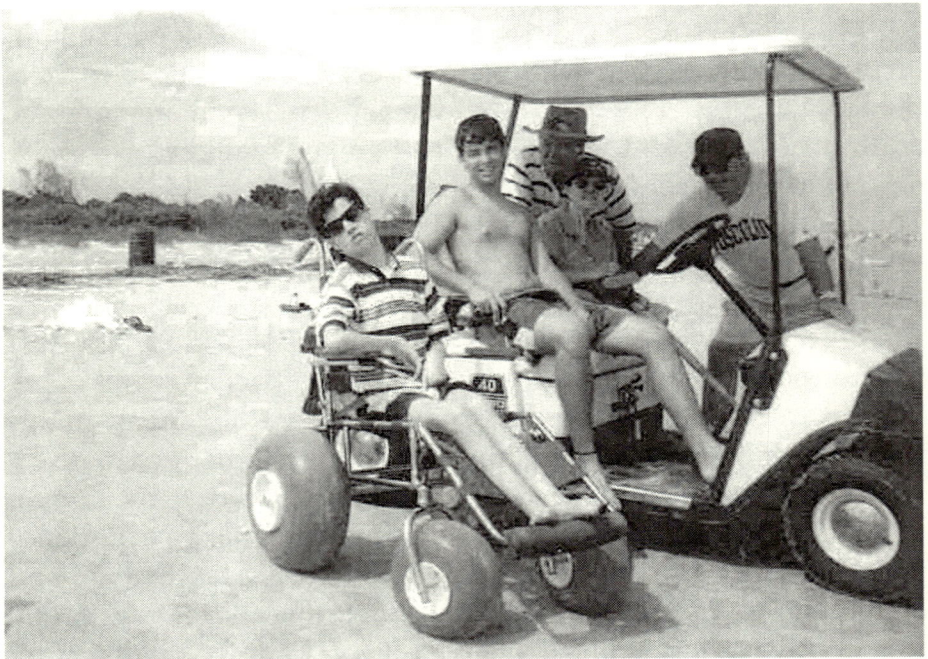

**Melany, Dad, Bill Taylor and sons Jonathan and Andrew
at St. Simons**

Some of our friends and family members from Augusta

came as did many family members from around that area. Her dad came from work and brought a friend and a co-worker who was saved that night as he was inspired by Melany's testimony and the message he heard from the stirring young preacher.

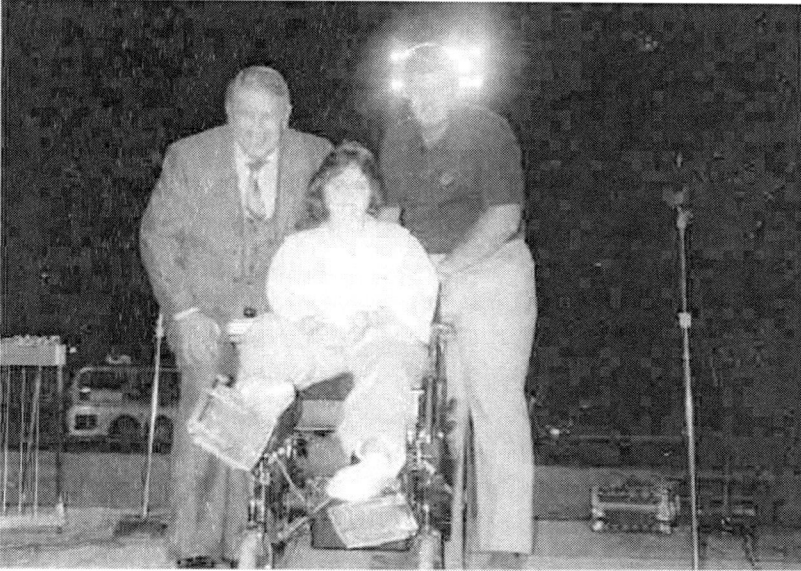

Melany with the Youth Rally speaker

Some of the college students who never went to church came to hear Melany and they were the ones I had talked to the Lord about when we were at Mayo. Remember, I had told Him how they could be moved by a small miracle because they had prayed so diligently for her.

Many of the young people were visibly touched by the things that Melany had to say and the radiance of her love for the Lord and others. The evangelist followed with a wonderful message.

At the close of the service we watched with great emotion and thanksgiving as young people left the bleachers and gathered on the football field for prayer -- and many to accept Jesus!

I thanked and praised the Lord. I knew He had answered

my prayer from Mayo though delayed it seemed to be to me, it was his own time. This was far better because these young people had now seen and heard from Melany what God had done for her and what He could do for them if they would only trust Him.

Praise be to God . . . he always answers our prayers! In her devotional book <u>*Streams in the Desert*</u> Mrs. Charles Cowman tells how the Children of Israel by faith sang and praised the Lord as they dug into the burning earth seeking much needed water. When they dug this well in the desert, they touched the stream that was running beneath, and reached the flowing tides that had long been out of sight.

She says, *"How beautiful the picture given, telling us of the river of blessing that flows all through our lives, and we have only to reach by faith and praise to find our wants supplied in the most barren desert.*

Our praise will still open fountains in the desert, when murmuring will only bring us judgment, and even prayer may fail to reach the fountain of blessing.

There is nothing that pleases the Lord so much as praise. There is no test of faith so true as the grace of thanksgiving. Are you praising God enough? Are you thanking Him for your actual blessings that are more than can be numbered, and are you daring to praise Him even for those trials which are but blessings in disguise? Have you learned to praise Him in advance for the things that have yet to come?"

Melany's college years continued to be very exciting and fun-filled. She was an officer in the FCA and made lifelong friends. She formed friendships and bonds with professors and counselors that she maintained all her life.

In 1987 Melany was first runner-up in the Miss Wheelchair of Georgia pageant in Albany, Georgia.

Several family members and some friends from college came for the pageant.

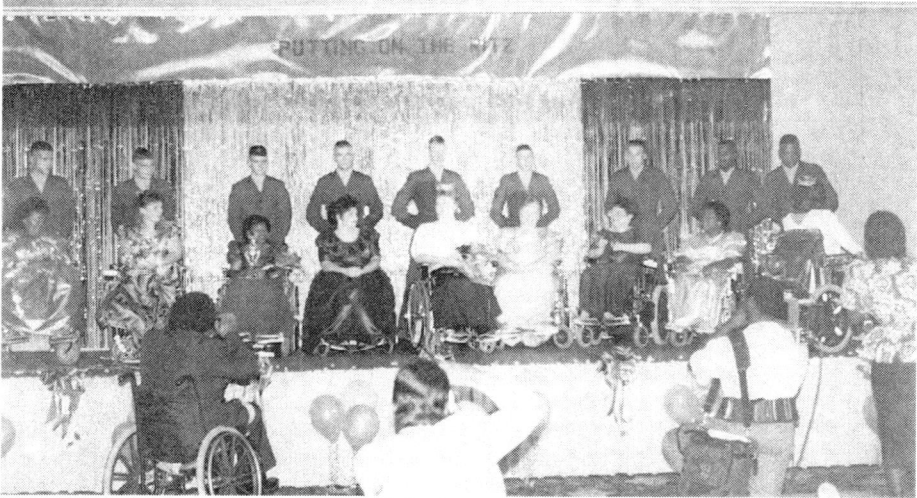

Miss Wheelchair Georgia Pageant

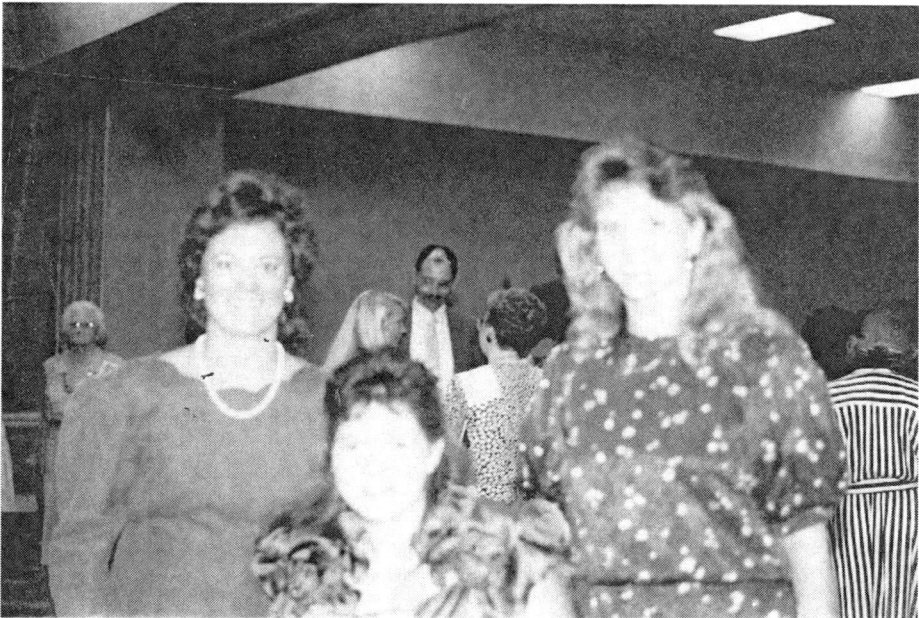

Becky, Melany and Mary at pageant

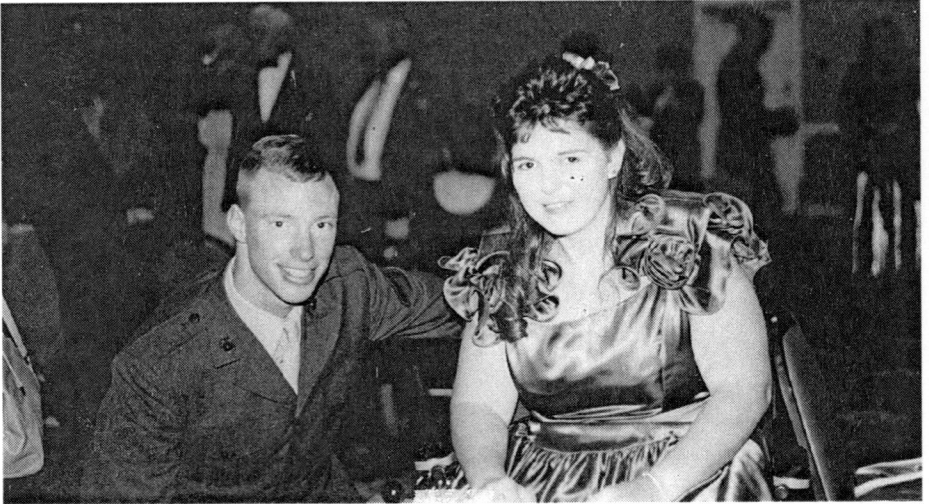
Melany and Escort at Miss Wheelchair Georgia

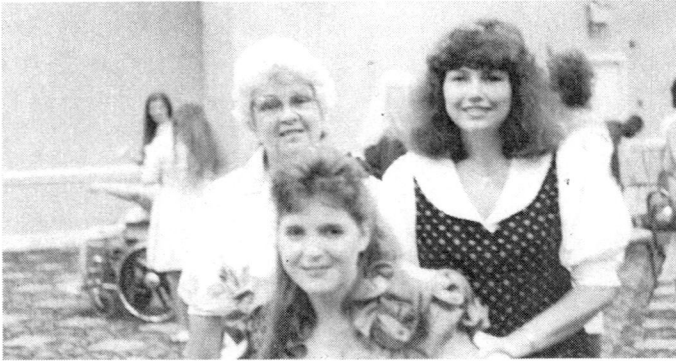
Melany with Aunt Sue and Cousin Pat at pageant

She was on the Dean's List every quarter. Also she received many honors and was inducted into the Phi Kappa Phi honor society and was honored by being included in several academic books, including *Who's Who of American College Students.*

It took her nine years to graduate. She always missed the winter quarter because of bronchitis and/or pneumonia. During those years she was in the hospital sixty times, totaling seven hundred and fifty days, according to hospital records.

Mary and Noel graduated in three years and the Lord sent

Dana, Rebecca, Pam, Lisa, Janet, and finally Terri as her roommates. They were all fine Christian girls and did a superb job of helping Melany with her needs. We continued paying those who were her actual caretakers because they had the major responsibilities.

The year before she graduated Melany was again in the hospital for almost a year. Her final year was very difficult health-wise but everyone supported. Finally it was time for Honors Day and graduation. Of course we went down for Honors Day. We all praised the Lord as she once again received many honors and accolades.

Two weekends before graduation Mel came home on Thursday and brought some of her accumulated stuff, also to attend her nephew's kindergarten graduation the following Monday.

On Friday morning I started to take Jake, my grandson, to kindergarten and my car would not start. Melany was already in her van to drive to the hospital for her Physical Therapy. We decided to ride together and Jake and I would drop her off at the hospital. I would take Jake to school and come back for her.

Melany drove about a block very slowly because children were walking to the bus stop. As we passed the stop she accelerated and the hand control malfunctioned. We had no brakes and the van continued to gain speed. As we reached the stop sign we went sailing across the very busy road at 8:30 a.m. Mel was cool and handled it very well. She was able to drive into a little lane on the other side of the road. We hit three trees and numerous logs before the van stopped. We praised the Lord that we did not hit a car. Jake's little head required twenty-five stitches. My leg was injured and Mel was unhurt.

Jake thought it was quite an adventure because we all went to the emergency room by ambulance. As we lay on stretchers reassuring each other that we were alright, the doctor sutured Jake's head. He told a nurse friend and James when he arrived

that we were three of the calmest wreck victims he had ever
seen. He said, "Even the baby didn't cry when I stitched his
head."

James said it was obvious the young doctor had no idea
what our life was like. An early morning wreck just started our
day of usual maladies.

Jake graduated from kindergarten on Monday with a huge
bandage on his head. Melany went back to college. My leg got
progressively worse and I wound up in the hospital with a deep
thrombosis in my groin.

I was kept very still with my legs elevated and my head
lowered slightly while they tried to dissolve the clot with blood
thinners.

As I have mentioned our family is very low-keyed and we
try to keep things in the right perspective.

An unusual thing happened on my third day in the hospital.
The chaplain who had visited Melany many times during her
many hospitalizations came into my room. He apologized for
not coming sooner, explaining he had been out of town. I told
him that was fine my own pastor had been daily and I did
appreciate him coming now.

He asked about Melany and about my condition and
inquired how I was handling the hospitalization. I reminded
him that I had told him a couple of years ago that my family,
especially Melany, did not only try to make the best of a bad
situation, but we always tried to see the good in the situation.

I explained that was exactly what I was doing. I had been so
busy with life that I had not had a lot of time to spend with God.
I had James bring my Bible and devotional book to the hospital,
as well as my daily prayer book, where I list and pray for needs
and record answers. I felt the Lord had given me this time of
meditation and prayer so that I could draw closer to Him. It had
been time well
spent.

The chaplain laughed and said he probably should not tell

me this, but one of the nurses on weekend duty who did not know me had asked him to come and visit me. She said a couple of the other nurses said even though I seemed alright and friendly, every time they came into the room I was lying with my eyes closed. The most significant thing they noticed was that I never had the television on.   They assumed if I wasn't interested in television I must be depressed. We both shared a laugh that it is a sad thing we live in such an electronic world today that something must be wrong with you if you don't want noises. I continued praying very diligently that I would be able to go to Melany's graduation.

Melany's friends and the Fletcher Memorial church members in Statesboro had helped her pack all week before graduation because I could not be there.   Also our friends Margaret and Joy from Augusta went to help her, as well as her friend Mary, and many other friends.

The doctors released me from the hospital on Friday morning. James, Ric, Jake and I went to Statesboro that afternoon and spent the night in a motel. I was in a wheelchair for the Saturday graduation and so thankful to be there.

What a wonderful day that was. We had one hundred-fifty friends and family members from out of town share in the glorious long awaited celebration and we all praised the Lord.

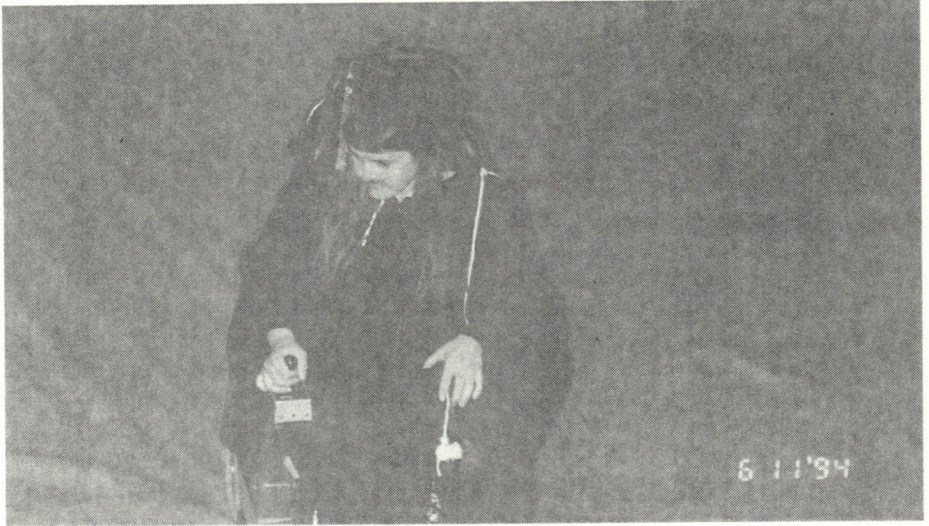

Melany at graduation

They built a ramp for Melany to get her motorized wheelchair on the platform. She was the first student at that time that had started to Southern in a wheelchair and graduated. She was the only one in her discipline that graduated Suma Cum Laude and the crowd cheered and gave her a standing ovation. We could not praise God enough!

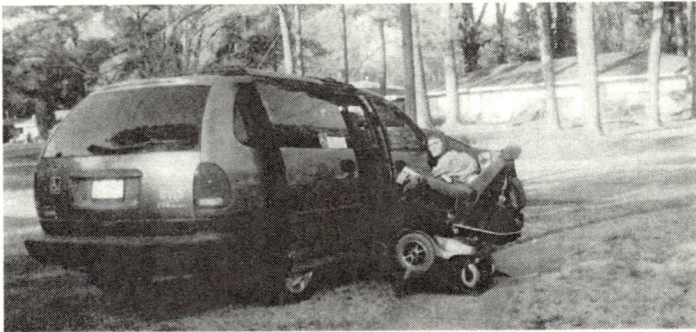

Graduation Present -- a new van!

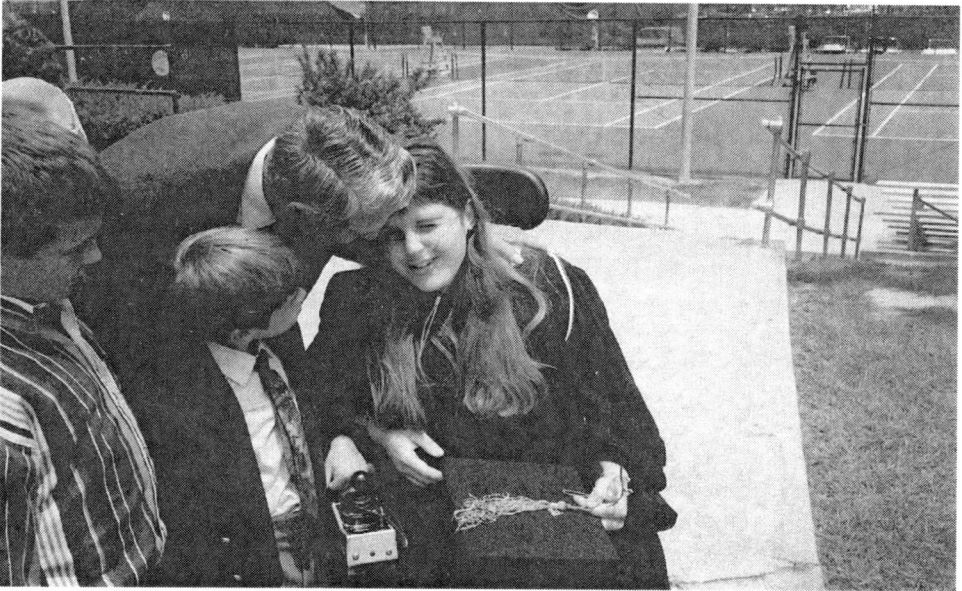

Melany with Uncle Decky, Scott and Jake

Melany's church in Statesboro, supervised by her cousin Barbara Patterson, had planned and taken care of the details for a lovely church reception. The church family took very good care of her as they had done during her college years.

Many of Melany's classmates, former classmates and their families came. Also, several of her professors and staff members attended. Everyone was so happy for her. She had made quite a lasting impression on the campus and the community.

One of her professors was a proclaimed agnostic. He told James and me what an impact Melany had made in his life. He said, "She is the only person I've ever met that inspired me to want to really know more about Jesus Christ." WOW!

Several others shared much about her life and her faith. It was a wonderful day for her and for all of us.

What grateful and sincere praises we raised to our Lord!

"He can take the life crushed by
Pain or sorrow and make it into
A harp whose music shall be all praise."
(J.R. Miller)
STREAMS IN THE DESERT

"When the fire of affliction
draws songs of praise from us,
Then indeed we are purified,
and our God is glorified."
STREAMS IN THE DESERT

CHAPTER IX
PRAISE CONTINUED

"His grace is sufficient for thee."
II Corinthians 12:9

Melany was so excited she had great plans for the summer. She planned to go to St. Simons Island to enjoy the summer and friends. She already had several offers for jobs in the fall.

She moved back home on Sunday, went into the hospital on Monday and stayed for several months. The doctors said she had used every bit of energy and stamina in pushing herself to complete her studies and graduate.

During this hospital stay she had four surgeries on her stomach and colon and one port-a-cath line replaced. They also changed her colostomy to an ileostomy which was much messier and more trouble to care for than a colostomy.

Once again she spent Thanksgiving, Christmas, her birthday and Easter in the hospital. She was asked once by an interviewer from the local newspaper how she endured being in the hospital for months or even a year at the time.

She replied, "Every time my door opened and someone came in, I saw them as a person with needs. Many had shared their needs and some had not. Whether it was a doctor, nurse, aide or housekeeper I tried to be friendly with them and prayed for them and their needs until the next person came in." This kept the focus off of herself and on others. So, she never got bogged down in her own pain and misery and self pity. She said, "I always praised God for the person and thanked Him for the service they rendered to me."

Is this not just what Jesus teaches us to do? Melany would

simply say, "I've submitted my entire life, prayer life and future to Christ and He will use me according to his will and plan."

When she was dismissed from the hospital after many months I went to the pharmacy to fill her prescriptions. They had removed more of her intestines and part of her stomach and the feeding supplement she had used several years could not be used any longer.

During the lengthy hospital stay the doctors had tried every type of feeding available. The only kind she could tolerate was a totally pre-digested feeding they used with premature babies. The surgeon told us he had heard it was expensive but he did not really know because he did not have a patient using it.

The clerk in the drug store rang up the feeding supplement and said it would be fifteen hundred dollars. I expressed my surprise as we had been paying one hundred-twenty five dollars per month for the other feeding. I said, "Oh, this is for several months supply?" She informed me that it was for one week. The feeding would cost six thousand dollars per month. Insurance nor Medicaid would pay for it because it was a feeding supplement and neither one covered that. When I got in the car, I cried all the way home.

When I told James he reassured me in his marvelous comforting way that with God's help we would work it out. We decided not to tell Melany because we knew it would worry her.

This was on Friday and on the Monday I called our insurance company and Medicaid. They both told me the same thing, they did not pay for feeding supplements. I called Melany's doctor. He felt so bad about our situation. He said not to worry, that this was not a supplement for Melany since now she could not eat anything so it was considered life sustaining.

Her doctor wrote a letter explaining Melany's situation. The companies still declined to pay. Six of her other doctors wrote similar letters. They still refused. However, they said that if she was in the hospital or we put her into a nursing facility they would pay for the feeding. They had paid for it while she was in the hospital. We could not put our child in a nursing home just so she could eat.

After several months of paying for Melany's feeding, I had contacted twenty-two different groups and agencies and was told we did not qualify for any type of aid or assistance. We fell through the cracks. We owned several rental houses that did not produce regular income. We owned a condo at the beach that was not paid for. On paper we had too many assets, but not enough cash flow to pay our bills and medical costs.

We started on a financial downhill spiral. We used all our resources of savings and most of our stocks and bonds. We refinanced our home and rental properties that we had already paid off and used all the money for her feeding, then every Friday I took James' entire pay check to the pharmacy. We had to depend on the unstable rental income to pay our household bills and to buy food. Most of the rent money went to pay the mortgage payments. We could not sell them because they were recently mortgaged.

Our son had a drug problem, so we had most of the expenses for our young grandson, who lived with us and had many needs.

We cut out all unnecessary spending and we barely survived. Of course Melany found out and felt so bad about the situation. We assured her that we did not mind the sacrifice, we were just so glad God spared her life and we had her. We all believed God would see us through this difficult time.

In thirty-six months we had paid over four hundred and eighty eight thousand dollars just for the feeding and several other medical expenses not covered by the insurance nor Medicaid.

During this time it was often difficult to continue praising God but we did. He is always worthy of our praise, regardless of circumstances.

We prayed constantly and we kept our faith in the Lord. Just when it looked like we were at the end of our proverbial rope, the Lord answered our prayers for financial relief.

They found a feeding that agreed with Melany that only cost two hundred dollars a week. We were ecstatic but it took a long time for us to catch up on our bills and to recover.

James had me keep a detailed account of our tithe during the time we simply could not pay it. That was the first main debt we paid.

True to His word just as the Lord did with Job, He restored most of what we had lost. It took us several years to completely recover. We continued our praise!

In October 1997 after Melany had again been in the hospital for several months the doctors were preparing to remove her colon and all but an eighth of her stomach. None of us were happy about this surgery, but it was necessary to save her life. Melany's brother was seven years older than she was, and she adored him. They were very close even though he had problems with drugs and alcohol intermittently for about ten years. Ric had gone into a rehabilitation center again and had been in recovery for a year. He was doing great and having a wonderful life. We were all so pleased, and of course we praised the Lord for the victory in his life.

Ric was working on a construction job near Richmond, Virginia, and would be returning to Augusta the first of November to work locally. He made double pay working on Saturday and Sunday so he would come home on Monday morning and leave on Tuesday evening.

He was quite concerned about not being here for Melany's surgery that was scheduled for Friday, October 24. She was only given a fifty per cent chance of living through the surgery but very little hope of life without it. It was a chance she was willing to take.

I stayed at the hospital most of the time because Melany was so ill. Ric had spent most of Monday afternoon with Melany until Jake came home from school then he went home to spend time with him and James. A friend came and stayed with Melany so I could go home and cook him his favorite meal Monday evening. Later I was so happy that I had done that. Ric came by on Tuesday afternoon as he was leaving town to see his sister.

Melany collected angels and had over two hundred that people had given her through the years. Ric brought her a small ceramic sitting angel that was blowing a kiss. He placed it on a high window ledge so she could see it from her bed. He said, "Mimi, I'm sorry Bubba can't be here Friday for your surgery. You just look at this little angel and know that wherever I am, I will be watching over you and praying for you." He kissed her and left.

I walked out to the front of the hospital where he was parked. He hugged and kissed me then started crying. and said, "Mother, please don't let Mimi die."

With heavy heart, I replied, "Son, I have always reminded you both to let your goodbyes be pleasant, and you always have. You never know what will happen in life. This well could be the last time that you see your sister here on earth." Then I added, "But, always remember, God's grace is always sufficient." These were the last words I said to my dear son. I wept as I watched him drive off in his prized purple Camaro. He went by the school to tell Jake goodbye and spent his second recess time with him.

Ric called his Dad when he got back to Virginia late Tuesday night. He called around eight o'clock Wednesday night and told his dad that he was tired and was going to bed soon. Sometime after that he called back and James must have been in the shower because he left a message on the answering machine. The hospital switchboard closed at nine o'clock so he often left me a message at home.

The message said he had picked some of the hot peppers he and Jake had planted in the back yard. He placed them in a large cooler cup and left them on his dresser. He asked me to send them to him so he could share them with his buddies. Then he said, "Mother, remember God's grace is always sufficient." These were the last words I heard my son say. He was killed at five-thirty the next morning on his way to work.

The last words I said to my son and the last words he said to me, "God's grace is always sufficient," has resounded in my heart and mind for many hours and days and still do today! Indeed, through the years God's grace is and has always been sufficient!

Ric had been killed in the early morning. The police did not get in touch with us until six o'clock that night. They had been to our home all day and would not tell our neighbors the reason. Finally our next door neighbor told them James was at work and I was at the hospital. I had gone home to get Jake ready for his football game. The head nurse called me and said that Melany was alright, but there was a policeman there and I needed to come back to the hospital immediately. James and Jake came home about that time and followed me to the hospital after Jake changed into his uniform, assuming he would be going on to his ballgame. The nice young police had already informed the nurses why he was there. The head nurse met me at the hospital entrance as we walked down the hall I sensed something was very wrong. I assumed it was concerning Melany because everyone was silent and some of the nurses at the station had tears in their eyes. They had called our assistant pastor (our pastor was out of town), and our good friends Joyce and Roy Scarborough. They took me into a conference room where they all were waiting seated at the long conference table. Melany's doctor and the hospital chaplain was there also. I remember feeling like ice water was running down my spine. They told me what happened. I can still recall the shock and horror I felt. It was unbelievable! When James and Jake arrived, Roy met them outside and took Jake to the snack bar while James came into the room. I will never forget how he literally crumpled sobbing with his face down on the long table.

Roy brought Jake in and we told him the Daddy that he worshipped had been killed. He was nine years old (ten in Dec.) and he tried to be so very brave. He had the presence of mind to ask the question that we had not asked, "Was anyone else hurt?"

The policeman explained to him about the accident. A lady in the car that had hit him was taken to the hospital but she had been released. Jake replied, "I'm glad about that. Are you really sure it was my dad and not someone else driving his car?" With tears in his eyes the officer he said they were sure. Jake wanted to go in to see Melany before he went home with Joyce and Roy.

One of the nurses had stayed with Melany while we were talking. She had told Melany I had been delayed in getting back and would be in soon. Melany was so sick she could hardly comprehend anything. Later she recalled when Dr. Jones came in and took her hand, followed by Jake, her dad and me on the other side of her bed, when she saw Pastor Dunn, the Chaplain, Joyce and Roy she knew something was very wrong. She said she could not understand why we had brought a police officer. She thought we had all come to tell her they were not going to be able to do the surgery and she was going to die. She said she wished it could have been her and not her beloved brother.

James and I stayed with her and the others left. Joyce had already called several of our friends who started arriving immediately. There was a library next to Melany's room and they filled it and the large waiting room. We were so grateful for the support they always gave us.

The doctors, nurses and staff at the hospital were wonderful to us as usual. We used the small library next to Melany's room to receive the many visitors for the next few days. On Sunday the day of the funeral they allowed us to use a large reception room for our church family to serve a meal for over one hundred and seventy of our family members and close friends.

Dr. Engler and Dr. Jones postponed Melany's surgery until Monday. They said they could not wait another day because of her serious condition. We were quite sad and very frightened.

Our funeral director Tommy King had been a friend of ours since high school. He had arranged to have Ric's body flown in Friday on a flight arriving at ten-thirty p.m.

A friend stayed with Melany as James and I went to the airport. What a different and difficult experience that was. We watched the family and friends wait by the outside gate in happy anticipation of welcoming those arriving, we stood farther down the portico with heavy hearts. We talked very little although we did speak of remembering the several times we had waited with joy to meet our son, sometimes in earlier days with his family.

The plane landed and taxied near the gate. We stood alone and wept as loved ones embraced. As the crowd dispersed we watched as the men finished unloading the baggage from the other side of the plane. Then we saw the hearse with the lights off slowly drive from the end of the runway to the other side of the plane. We moved farther down the walk to watch as we saw them bring a large wooden box off and load it in the back of the hearse. We sobbed as we hastened to our car to follow the hearse to the funeral home.

We rode in silence several miles down the highway behind the hearse. Then James said brokenly, "One of the dearest treasures God has let us have was unloaded in a wooden box, hidden and treated like a thief in the night." I'm sure it must need to be handled like that because some people probably would not be comfortable knowing there was a dead body on the plane.

We watched from the lane that led to the back of the funeral home as they took that precious body of our dear son inside.

One of the few times in my life I was speechless. We drove in silence back to the hospital. We went into the empty lobby and James led me to a couch and we sat down. He took me in his loving arms and we cried. Then he said, "We must continue praying, because without God's help and the deep love we have for each other and for Melany and Jake I don't know how we can make it through these next few days." I still could not speak.

Then he prayed and poured out his heart to the Lord. He concluded his prayer thanking and praising God for giving us these wonderful children to enjoy and love and asking Him to give us strength in the coming days and to please let Melany survive the surgery.

Family members began arriving from out of town Saturday, including Jake's mother, Charlotte. They came by the hospital to visit with Melany before going to the viewing. Our friends were there all day helping us in any way they could. Two friends stayed with Melany while we went to the funeral home that night. Her dear friend Stan Brassell made pictures of the flowers there. My cousin Pam videotaped the viewing for Melany.

The funeral service was led by our pastors John Bryan and Sherrell Dunn. Ric's Sunday School teacher Marie Wilson sang, as well as our longtime friend Joanne Farr. Jake's band director, Phil Brewer played the trumpet concluding a beautiful service. Melany and Ric's former youth director, Tom Lowry videotaped the entire service for her.

My anguished heart had many questions--but few answers.

Ruth Graham describes my heart cry in her poem (Sitting By My Laughing Fire).

My Son

"How can I pray while my heart cries,
'You killed my son?'
What can I say?
How look for comfort from
the one who willed it done?
Omnipotent, He could have
stopped it if He would!
My son---My son---
Numb with grief,
My soul is one vast 'Why?'
His life was all too brief;

He was so young to die.
Where were you Lord?
Where were you?
Gently He replied,
"Just where I was dearly, dearly loved,
When mine was crucified.'"

Ruth Bell Graham

Many of our family members from out of town stayed for Melany's surgery the following day. She was in intensive care for several days and was very sick for several months.

Melany was finally able to go home without the expensive tube feeding because they had removed most of her stomach. The tube now went into the Jejunum, a section of the small intestine.

Melany missed her brother a lot especially after she was able to go home. Ric and Jake had lived with us since Jake was three years old after Ric & Charlotte had divorced. He was more like a little brother to her than a nephew. They enjoyed each other very much.

Melany had only been home a few days when Jake became very sick. The doctor treated him for a stomach virus that was later diagnosed as appendicitis. His appendix ruptured and they performed emergency surgery on him the night of February twelfth. He was very ill and two days later he developed double pneumonia and almost died. We were so grateful to God for sparing his life.

Jake's classmates all wrote him delightful and often funny notes of good wishes. When he was able to receive visitors his teacher brought the entire class to visit and they brought small gifts. We were thankful for such a caring teacher and young people.

Our family unit remained strong. Through the years when James and I faced any problems, severe illnesses, or even death we just bonded closer physically, emotionally and spiritually.

That got us through some very difficult times. We still had great support in family and friends.

James retired in April 1998 so he could help me more with Melany and Jake. We felt it was very important for Jake to be able to continue the sports (football, basketball, baseball and table tennis) that he enjoyed so much. Although all these sports had seasons they all demanded a good bit of time in practices and attending games. Ric had been a tremendous help with this.

We all missed Ric daily and we tried to keep his memory alive for Jake. James and I both have first cousins whose dads died suddenly when they were twelve years old. Neither remembers anything about their dads and they encouraged us to help Jake remember things he shared with Ric. They both agreed losing their dads so young had apparently been so traumatic and painful they could not remember anything good or bad about them. We talked openly as the occasion arose and let Jake talk and share things he remembered.

When he was twelve years old he wrote the following poem about his dad. Years later he said Fathers Day was more difficult for him than any other holiday. I have shared this poem (with his permission) with several fathers because it reminds us of the things our children and grandchildren really remember when we are gone. It is the time given to them and not the material things we try to give.

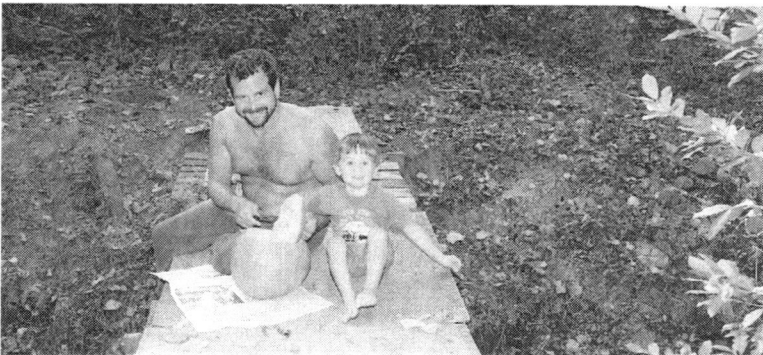

Ric and Jake carving a pumpkin

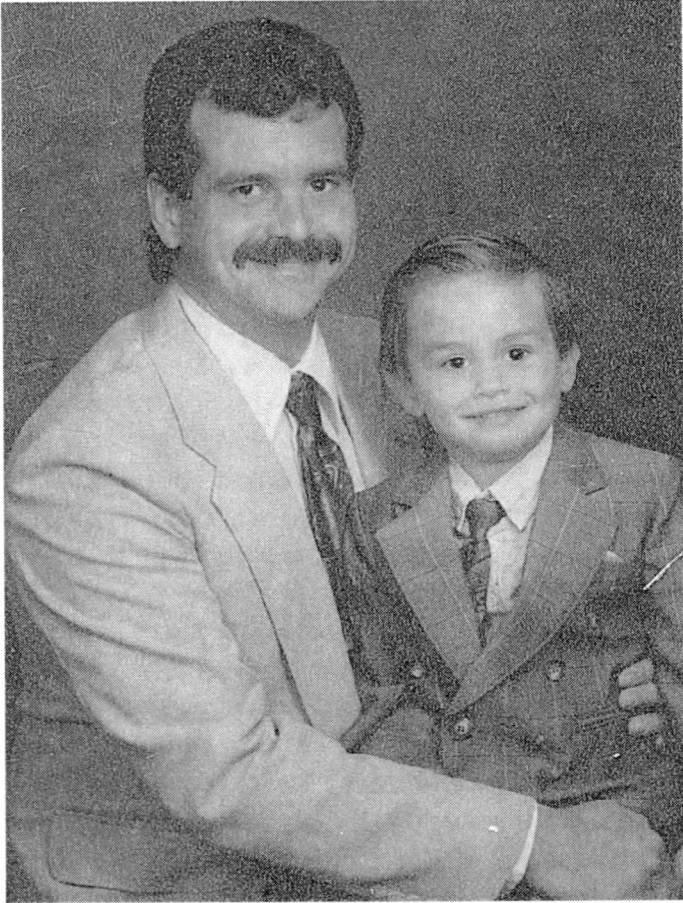

Ric and Jake

"I REMEMBER"
Well Dad, it's Father's Day again,
My friends gave cards to their dads saying how great they are;
I had a hard time finding a card to put on your crypt,
Saying what a good dad you were and how
much you mean to me;
I REMEMBER HOW GREAT YOU WERE.

My friends went to church with their dads and families,
I went with my Papa and Nana;
I looked at the picture hanging on my bedroom wall,

Of you and me and Mommie made at church when you dedicated me;
I REMEMBER GOING TO CHURCH WITH YOU.

My friends took their dads out for lunch,
I went with my grandparents to your favorite restaurant; I ordered the
"Ultimate Feast"--just like we used to, But it didn't taste the same
without you;
I REMEMBER EATING OUT WITH YOU.

My friends gave their dads gifts for Father's Day,
I'm sure I was the only one who had to take a flower arrangement to the
cemetery;
I REMEMBER HOW YOU ALWAYS "Made over" the countless
little "Junkie stuff" I picked out and gave you for your day.

My friends spent the afternoon playing ball or just hanging out with
their dads,
I went to the cemetery and took your card and Flowers.
I REMEMBER THE GOOD TIMES WE HAD.

I REMEMBER HOW PROUD YOU WERE:
I could play video games at age 2
I could read at age 4
I caught my first fish
I learned to ride my bike
I hit my first homerun
I got my first touchdown

I REMEMBER:
How kind you were to me and to others
How you cried when Mimi was in pain
How you laughed
How your cologne smelled
How you always had time to play with me
How we always had a great time together
How we had long talks about everything
I REMEMBER HOW QUICKLY YOU LEFT ME!

Well Dad, another Father's Day is over,
As my friends think of the great day they had with
their dad;
I think about you and how much I miss you,

And I wonder--WILL I ALWAYS BE ABLE TO REMEMBER?
I PRAY THAT I WILL!!!

The plaque that we had placed on Ric's crypt was very befitting, it simply reads:

Too well loved,
To ever be forgotten.

Jake with his first fish

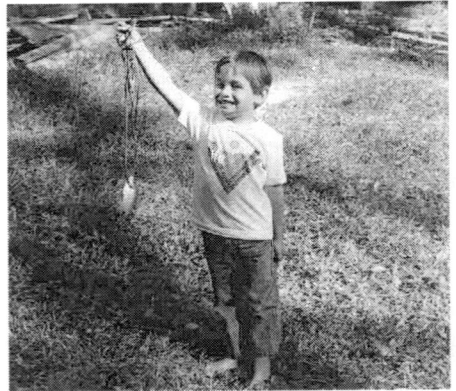

Jake still enjoys sharing things he remembers about his dad, looking at pictures of him and the stories we share with him about his dad, especially when he was young.

In May nineteen-ninety eight they had to remove Melany's legs above the knees. One had been drawn up for about ten years and the other one for about four years. It was very difficult to lift her because her hips would come out of their sockets when you lifted her legs. Also she had several blood clots (emboli) because of the lack of circulation.

The wonderful orthopedic doctor, Dr. Edward Crosland

really hated to do this but it was necessary. After healing from the surgery it was so much easier to move and transport her. Most of the time she could transfer herself now. Her doctor told me one day, with tears in his eyes that she was really a remarkable young woman. He said he had never had anyone thank him for removing their legs and making their life easier. She always was remarkable!

Melany made the statement one day, "Well, I guess now I really will never walk again. I guess you can give my skateboard, bicycle, pogo stick and skates away." She had been in a wheelchair for eighteen years but she still had hopes of walking again. She continued praising the Lord that she could transfer herself again since her legs had been removed.

We were doing well financially but we did not have the assets we had in the past. James prayed intently that the Lord would somehow help us to return to the place we could have enough money to take care of Melany and leave enough to care for her and Jake when we were no longer on this earth or if we had another financial disaster.

The Lord provided us with a marvelous opportunity to invest in a new company. Canada had just lifted the restrictions on their automatic teller machines. They were allowing them to be placed in most of the places that American ATM Machines are in, instead of just being connected with banks. In 1999 James took my dear nephew Lamar with him to Canada and they invested in machines and started a new company called E-Cash Systems.

Lamar had worked in the ATM business in Georgia. He was very knowledgeable and qualified to teach the Canadian people how to sell the machine concept and install them in businesses. Then we would receive the residuals from each machine.   Plus James said with his personality and ability Lamar could sell anything to anyone.

They had a wonderful fun-filled and quite profitable time.

James stayed for a couple of years, coming home most weekends (every one, if Jake had a ballgame, or we had a real need).

Lamar still has the business in Canada which has changed names several times. He has had several ups and downs, he has handled them in a positive way. James would be proud of him today and his accomplishments. Lamar now has a satellite office in Georgia that allows him and his precious Canadian wife, Marg to be in the states several months each year.

God always provides when we trust and honor Him, and give Him the continual praises He deserves!

"Weeping inconsolably beside a grave can never give back love's banished treasure,
Nor can any blessing come out of such sadness.
We really never get over our great griefs;
We are never altogether the same after we have passed through them as we were before."
STREAMS IN THE DESERT

"The joy set before us should shine upon our griefs as the sun shines through the clouds, glorifying them.
God has so ordered, that in pressing on in duty, we shall find the truest, richest comfort for ourselves."
STREAMS IN THE DESERT

CHAPTER X
PEACE

My own peace I give you."
John 14:27 (Weymouth)

Melany loved children and by this time in her life (early thirties) most of her friends were married with children. She thoroughly enjoyed the children visiting and playing with them. She developed a blood disorder and her white count dropped very low. The doctors feared her getting any infection because they had used all the available places to put a port-a-cath line, as the previous lines would get infected or just clot off. Finally the thoracic surgeon, Dr. Michael Watts, had placed the line directly into her heart, a first time procedure according to the available records. It worked well but her physicians felt she should stay out of crowds and away from small children.

We would shop with her after ten o'clock and sometimes after midnight to avoid the crowds. She was so disappointed not to be able to see the children or hold a precious baby. I said, "Lord did this little thing that brought her such great pleasure have to be taken from her as well?" He answered not a word but again I heard the resounding words, "My grace is always sufficient." Melany's dream of one day being able to work with children in a hospital using her many hours of preparation would never be. She had committed her life to be used in this vocation or mission work or wherever God wanted to use her. It is hard to give up a worthy dream but she attained complete peace.

We began to see a calmness come over her attitude and spirit. She had committed many things and painful situations to the Lord in prayer she was now at peace for the Lord to use her anyway He desired for His glory.

Watching her life we were reminded of a poem by Mrs. Charles Cowman:

> *There is a peace that cometh after sorrow,*
> *Of hope surrendered, not of hope fulfilled;*
> *A peace that looketh not upon tomorrow,*
> *But calmly on a tempest that is stilled.*
>
> *A peace that lives not now in joy's excesses,*
> *Nor in the happy life of love secure;*
> *But in the unerring strength the heart possesses,*
> *Of conflicts won while learning to endure.*
>
> *A peace there is, in sacrifice secluded,*
> *A life subdued, from will and passion free;*
> *'Tis not the peace that over Eden brooded,*
> *But that which triumphed in Gethesmane.*

One afternoon James and I were sitting in the swing out by our backyard creek. James said, "I don't know how to tell you this, but the Lord has laid on my heart that He is not going to heal Melany but continue to use her condition for His Glory." I started to cry, because God had laid the same thoughts on my heart and mind several days ago and I had not told anyone. In a few minutes Jake came to the back door and said, "Mimi wants us to come to her room she wants to talk with us."

Melany said, "I don't know how to tell you this, but I want you to stop praying for the Lord to heal me. Just use your prayers for sustaining grace for me, and pray for others. God has laid on my heart," (almost identical words He had given to me and James), "He is not going to heal me, but use my condition for His glory. Pray that I'll allow this to happen in my life. I want to be in his will and a blessing to others."

James and I immediately looked at a framed poem that someone had given to her. It hung over her desk. It said:

*There has never been known great
saintliness of soul
which did not pass through great suffering.*

*When the suffering soul reaches
a calm sweet carelessness,
When it can inwardly smile at its own suffering
and does not even ask God
to deliver it from suffering.
Then it has wrought its blessed ministry.
Then patience has its perfect work;*

*Then the crucifixion begins
to weave itself into a crown."*

Author unknown

When Melany had graduated from college, one of the counselors, Audrey Campbell who had been close to her for entire nine years of college gave her this framed poem. What a blessing Audrey was to Melany and to our entire family, she visited us often at home and she and Melany remained "close hearts" until Melany's death.

The Lord still used Melany in wondrous ways. She started making grapevine wreaths with natural sea shells she had gathered on our many trips to the beach. She included a small angel or cherub on each one and added beautiful ribbons and bows. Each had a little handmade card on with a stamped gold angel. "Lovingly handcrafted by Mimi," and *"For He shall give His Angels charge over thee in all thy ways."* Psalm 91:11 was printed on the card including her phone number. These were sold at craft stores and she had many calls for individual orders. She gave many as gifts as well.

People called and expressed appreciation for the Bible Verse and she was given the opportunity to witness of God's care and love. She never failed to explain the way of salvation and the certainty of our living in Heaven forever when we accept Jesus as our Savior if the time was right. She didn't push her belief or faith, she simply lived it and shared it with others if they were interested.

Melany had a small sitting room adjacent to her bedroom where she could have privacy when her guests came if she was able to sit up. A craft room joined the sitting room. Her supplies were on a large table where she worked anytime she was physically able. She enjoyed this very much.

The next few years had a remarkable sameness. Melany had to spend more time in the house and the bed because of the pain in her back and her weakening condition.

She was still able to drive occasionally and was a very safe and careful driver. Her driving mainly consisted of a five mile radius, the doctors' offices, the hospital where her Huber needle was changed each week, the drugstore, and the beauty shop. Occasionally she was able to go to church and the mall accompanied by someone. It gave her a real feeling of independence and pleasure.

We continued going to the beach for two months each year. The last time we drove to St. Simons the trip took us twelve hours instead of five. We had to stop often because her pain was so intense we could not ride more than fifteen to twenty miles at the time. We flew her back home and continued flying her back and forth after that.

Noel and Julie, former roommates, lived on the island with their families. The girls spent a lot of quality time together. Their husbands Jim and Ken were so sweet to keep the children and make this time possible. Often during the day the girls would bring their children to the beach, pool or playground at the pier. The girls would visit and Melany could see the children in the open air but not get close to them. It seemed she always had to be on the outside, looking in at someone else's joy, but she never complained. We had decided years before she always took her own sunshine wherever she went and she created her own joy!

We enjoyed our grandson Jake immensely and home schooled him the two months we were at the beach each year. It was amazing how much Jake looked like his dad, however he had a lot of Melany's ideas and expressions and they were very close.

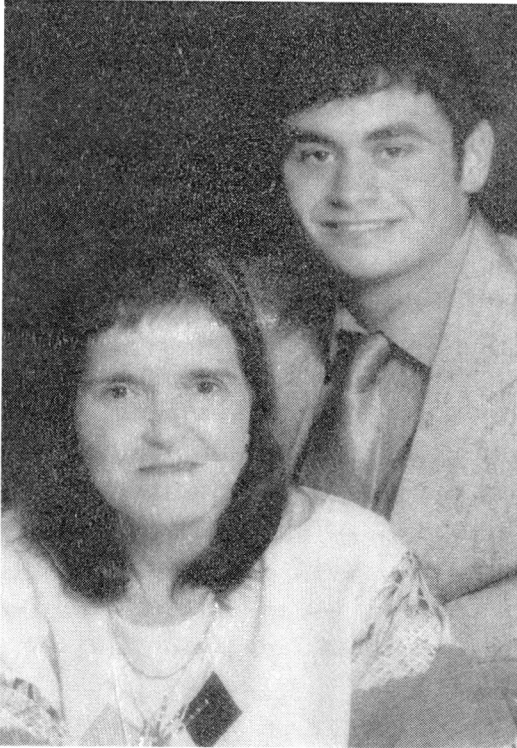

Jake with Melany in 2004

Melany particularly enjoyed one of the episodes with Jake when he was about seven or eight years old. He talked back to me which was very unusual for him. I patiently reminded him that I did not allow this and he would have to be punished.

He said, "Nana, I don't know what happened. My mind told me I had better stop, but my mouth just kept going." That sounded like something Melany would have said at that age. I told him I did understand we all had times our mouth ran away with us but we needed to practice controlling it.

Melany was in the hospital many more times. In 2000 the surgeon removed the end of her spine (a coccygectomy and partial sacretomy). She could sit up a little longer and could attend several of Jake's sports events.

Jake played football and baseball for our recreation department until he was in middle school. He was able then to play those sports as well as basketball and table tennis and was on the tennis team for the school. Melany enjoyed attending a few of his games. Young people are wonderful and so energetic and we enjoyed his friends in our home.

We went to a house at the lake twenty miles away for a couple of weeks each year. We always took friends of Jake and Melany. Once we had six extra boys and two of Melany's friends in a three bedroom house. That was a house full!

We have a pontoon boat that the electric wheelchair could drive on easily. Melany loved to fish from the boat and we all enjoyed going out for the gorgeous sunsets.

When Jake finished grade school, we had his entire class of boys and girls at the lake for a "graduation" (end of the year) party. We had rented an additional house so we could separate the boys and girls. Jake and Melany both came down with the chicken pox, exposing all the others. Some of the parents were very unhappy, because they had planned to leave shortly after school for vacation.

James came home from Canada for several months. In February 2001 he suffered a massive heart attack. He almost died and had to have triple bypass surgery. Jake attended the same church school his dad and Melany had attended. One of the mothers came and took Jake to his basketball game after I had taken James to the hospital.

The young people called James, Papa and he was their number one fan and supporter. When the boys received the news of his heart attack they all circled the court in the gym and prayed for him. We were grateful for the people of all ages who have prayed for us through many difficult situations. James had never been sick before. He was very strong and had a complete recovery.

Things were going rather calm and peacefully. A letter arrived informing us that when James retired and started receiving Medicare Melany should have been put on Medicare because she had been disabled as a child. This started numerous phone calls and letters because with Medicare she had no prescription coverage. Also, she had capped out her total of one million dollars on the hospital and pharmacy insurance She would always max out her yearly cap, which is what would help to put us in such a difficult financial situation before. But now this was permanent.

One medicine was $9,000 per month and her total pharmacy bill was around $15,000 per month. Our only regular income was from our Social Security and a pension retirement. We had the income from Canada although the amount was not consistent.

We informed them we had followed all the guidelines since her college graduation. We were told if she had a private room with a lock on the door, her own bathroom, and paid us $200 per month out of her small SSI check, she was considered as a head of household of one and could always get the medical coverage, Medicaid and a small disability check.

The rules had changed and no one told us. We had gone through the proper channels in applying for Social Security for me and James two years earlier when he reached retirement age. They knew we had a disabled daughter but somehow a clerical error was made. They said since it was their mistake we would probably not be required to repay the two years of services she had been given erroneously.

That would have been around $900,000 for the medicines

plus three extended hospital stays and regular doctor visits. It would have been well over a million dollars. We were grateful we did not have to pay this back as it would have been impossible.

Many people tried to help us including our doctors and our pastor. Politicians from both political parties set agendas aside and tried to work together. Finally we were able to get a temporary relief. We had paid $15,000 per month until once again we were getting in financial difficulties. We trusted in the Lord and had a peace that He would help us work it out.

The Lord provided a wonderful solution for us. We went to the beach for November and December 2002 because our unit was not rented. While there we found all beach front property had become quite valuable. We had a prime beachfront condo and were offered a very good price for it. The young entrepreneur and his family had become very close to our family and especially to Melany since his wife had several medical needs. As part of the deal we could use the condo for two months each year as long as it was not during prime rental time. What a blessing! We prayed about it and decided to sell it and then purchase two condos (we actually purchased three) in Augusta that we had seen.

In July 2003 we closed on the beach property. In February 2004 they finished building our three condos and we moved in. We had a door cut between two of them. James and I lived in one side and Jake on the other. That gave Jake and his friends a large living room, complete with TV, pool table, video games and all his sports trophies displayed in a cabinet. He had his own kitchen for snacks and soft drinks and a large bedroom and large bath. I used his guest bedroom for my office, where I could keep an eye on things, especially when girls visited. The best part for James and me was closing the door on the teenagers mess and noises! We loved young people but we needed a little peace and quiet and privacy sometimes.

James called the condos "doll houses" but we enjoyed our small one. We had a guest room and he especially enjoyed not having yard work! With the three condos we had twelve rooms which was the same number from our previous home. We now had six bathrooms and three kitchens that I was responsible for cleaning instead of the one kitchen and three bathrooms we had previously. I wasn't sure who had the better deal, when I would laughingly tell this to our friends, James said, "Well, this is what you wanted." That was very true.

Melany was totally ecstatic. She had dreamed since college graduation of having her own place. She was especially grateful to our builder, Dusty Caron. He as many others had done, went far above his duty and responsibility in trying to make Melany's condo just as she wanted it. She was able to pick out the furnishings and she had a guest room for her friends to stay overnight.

She had curio cabinets to display over three hundred angels given to her by friends, family and acquaintances. It was a beautiful reminder of God's watchcare over us all.

We had a small lake that came right up to our back patios. We enjoyed sitting out, watching the many birds in the wetland across the lake and the sunsets were spectacular and peaceful.

Now Melany was head of household of one, and all of her financial benefits were restored and should not be taken away again. We were so thankful for God's goodness to us.

One of the most enjoyable things for Melany was fishing from her backyard which she really loved. But as happened so often with Melany her enjoyment was short lived. J.R. Miller describes this in an article:

Must life be a failure for one compelled to stand still in enforced inaction and see the great throbbing tides of life go by? No, victory is then to be gotten by standing still, by quiet waiting. It is a thousand times harder to do this than it was in the active days to rush on in the columns of stirring life. It requires a grander heroism to stand and wait and not lose heart and not lose hope, to submit to the will of God, to give up work and honors to others, to be quiet, confident and rejoicing, while the happy, busy multitude go on and away. It is the grandest life "having done all, to stand."

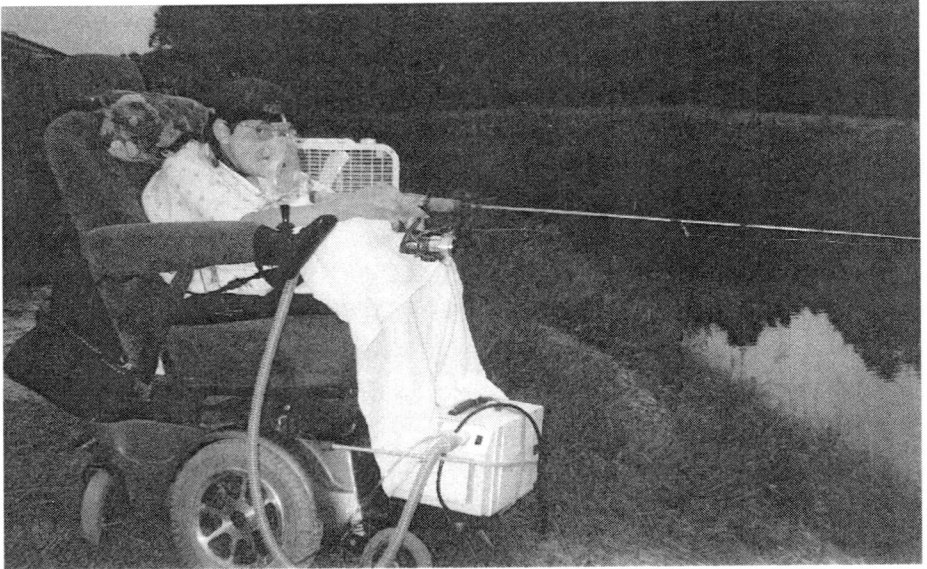

Melany fishing

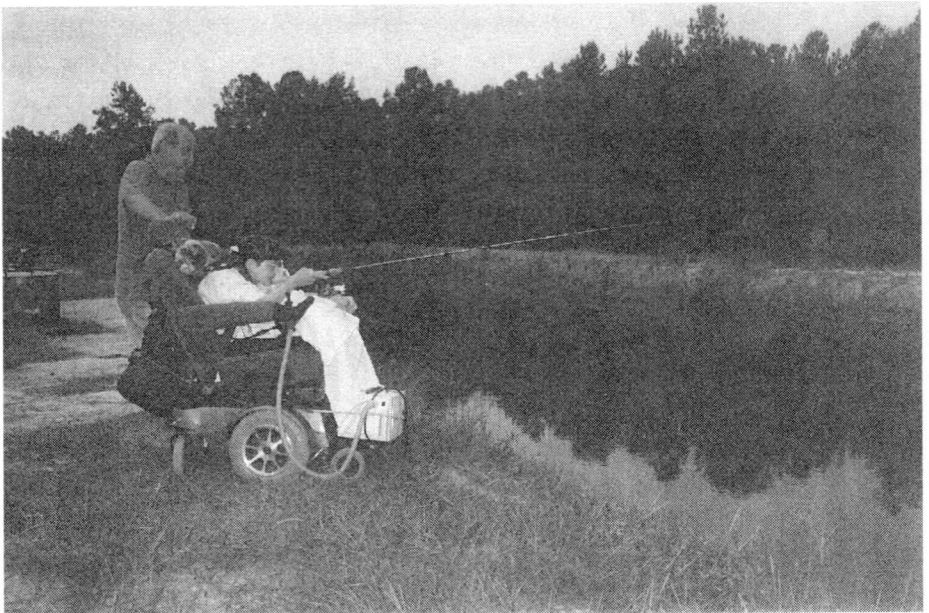

Dad James and Melany fishing

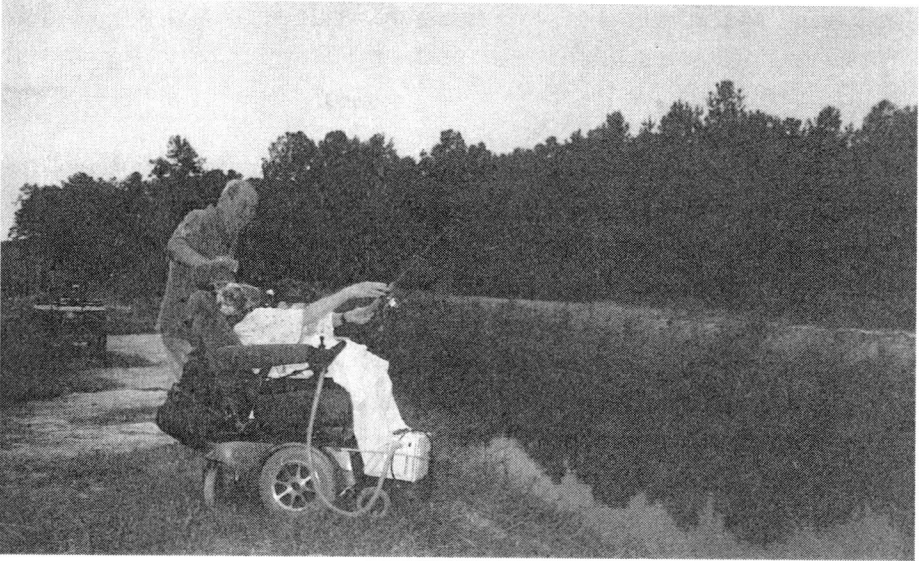

Reeling in a catch (above); Melany with James and catfish (below)

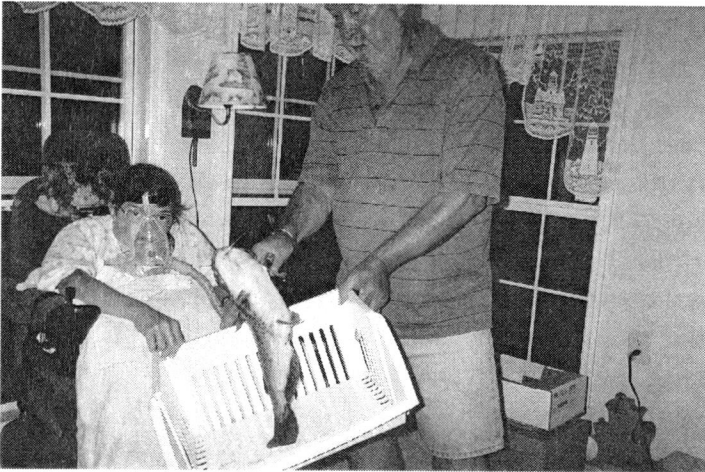

It really seemed every time things were going well for her, everything crashed. She had two months of independence and bliss, enjoying her condo, sitting on her patio with her little poodle, Tico, fishing everyday and staying alone. All the condos were handicapped accessible so she could move around easily in all of them.

Then much of her enjoyment ended.   Many of her supporting muscles had weakened and some had deteriorated from the ravaging of the Behcets. Her hip muscles were getting very painful and weak.

One day as she bent over from her wheelchair to pick up her little dog her hip became dislocated. The pain was unreal! The orthopedic doctor advised complete bed rest for at least eight weeks. He said the hip would probably work back into the socket as the irritated nerves settled down. He said it might continue to happen because there was very little muscle support to hold it in place. They decided a hip replacement would not work because of the condition of the supporting muscles. She patiently endured the pain and the confinement although it was beautiful spring weather, perfect for fishing.

The first day she was out of bed, I took her to the beauty shop for a shampoo. As the beautician let the chair back for the shampoo it became stuck. She pushed hard on the back of it and the chair turned over on top of Melany. I could tell the pain was excruciating and the hip had come out of its socket again, because we heard a snap.

Everyone was so sweet and helpful to her. The owner of the shop insisted we call the EMTS. Melany said no, she just wanted to go home. I assured the owner she would be alright and as Christians we did not believe in suing. We did not realize the "snap" we heard was actually the bone in the short nub of her leg cracking. Her beautician who had been her friend since high school was hysterical and her husband was called to come and drive her home.

Melany always tried to put people at ease in times like these. She said, "Please do not feel bad. I have been dropped in better places than this, such as church, school and public places. My dad and brother dropped me down the side of a mountain path one time, and I'm still here. Don't worry about it, it was simply an accident."

In spite of her brave announcement, I knew she was in

terrific pain. At home she began another painful five months of complete bed rest. Her body deteriorated rapidly, but not her attitudes or her spirits.

Everyone observed as one of her often repeated Bible verses came into fruition.

II Corinthians 4:16b says, *"Though our outward man perish, yet the inward man is renewed day by day."*

We all witnessed as her body seemed to waste away, her inward self was indeed renewed in complete peace.

> "Why must I weep when others sing?
> 'To test the deeps of suffering.'
> Why must I work while others rest?
> 'To spend my strength at God's request?'
> Why must I lose while others gain?
> 'To understand defeats sharp pain!'
> Why must this lot of life be mine
> When that which fairer seems is thine?
> 'Because God knows what plans for me
> Shall blossom in eternity.'
> **STREAMS IN THE DESERT**

CHAPTER XI
PEACE PREVAILS

"And the peace of God, which passeth all understanding,
shall keep your hearts and minds through Christ Jesus."
Philippians 4:7

Melany's pain was unreal from April 2004 through April 2005 and then became excruciating and almost unbearable. The strong pain medicine given every two hours would help her sleep for about an hour and a half, then the pain was awful for the thirty minutes until she could have the strong medication again.

Melany had spent many happy uplifting hours talking with friends and family. This was very difficult for all of us but her peace was so remarkable. We recognized and agreed she was simply tired of struggling every day just to stay alive even in pain.

We watched with heavy hearts as we realized Melany had lost most of the quality of her life. Her nubs were drawing up against her chest with severe spasms. She still did not complain.

Melany always enjoyed visits and phone calls but she was becoming very tired and weak. There were many times family and friends called to come for a visit and she was just to weak to see them, or even to talk on the phone with them.

On Tuesday June 7, 2005, Melany made the decision with her doctor to go into Hospice- Palliative Care at St. Joseph. They hoped that they could help her control her pain with pain management. Her pain was so great she would pray aloud and beg the Lord for enough relief to be able to use the bedpan. It would break our hearts that God did not grant this seemingly small and simple request.

The doctors tried several medications but even with the increased Buprenex the awful pain in her nubs and back continued. Melany was getting weaker and weaker. She was so ill and tired.

One Sunday morning we were watching our Pastor, Mark Harris on television. He was talking about the white cloud in Revelation 4:10. He said just as Christ ascended into Heaven in a white cloud, one day He will return for us in a white cloud. I didn't even think Melany was aware of what was being said.

As Melany opened her eyes she motioned for me to come closer to her bed. She said, "Mom, please call Mark and ask him to ask Jesus to please bring the white cloud right here outside my window and take me to Heaven with Him. I want to go to Heaven so badly, I'm so tired."

Many times I have definitely felt the Lord's direction very clear and plain. However there have been several times I felt certain the Lord was guiding me and it did not work out as I thought it would or should. While Melany was in the hospital I had prayed long and hard for her pain to be relieved. As I wrote in Chapter VII about being at Mayo, I remembered they were experimenting with Botox to try to relieve severe muscle spasms.

The doctors talked with us about trying it with Melany the night before we were to come back home to Georgia. I had spoken with a physician friend about it and he said it was experimental.

We felt that she was too weak to have a trial done which would require staying two more weeks. James had chartered the air ambulance and was coming the next day to get us and we were ready to go home. When they told us it was a type of poison we definitely decided against it.

I had completely forgotten about Botox even though in the ensuing twenty plus years it had become a very widely used and sought after medication with many uses. I told Melany about it and she said this was unreal. She had cleaned out her wallet before she came into the hosptal. She had found a card that had been given to her years before about a doctor at Medical College that was working with Botox for muscle spasms.

We felt it had been directed by God because we called and learned a doctor we knew at The Medical College of Georgia (MCG) was now using Botox for children with Cerebral Palsy and some with Muscular Dystrophy. They were also injecting some adults who had Multiple Sclerosis. Botox relieved the severe muscle spasms and spasticity associated with these diseases.

Melany's doctor called and arranged for her to be seen by Dr. Rivener, the Botox Specialist. James and I accompanied her by ambulance to MCG. We had great expectations that this could help her. The doctor checked Melany, studied her records and said with her difficult situation she would not be a good candidate for the Botox Treatment. In her case it would involve using very long needles inserted through her abdomen into the nerves in her spine. He felt she was too sick and her condition was too delicate to be used as a guinea pig. Her nubs were still drawn up to her chest and in constant motion with the very painful spasms. She was so sick that she was unaware most of the time. James and I both wept as we stood at the head of Melany's bed so she could not see us.

Dr. Rivener said a doctor at MCG had perfected a surgical procedure called a Laminectomy, in layman's terms, a nerve-muscle lobotomy. Neurosurgeon, Dr. Haroon Choudhri would go into the spinal column and Dr. Rivener would use the nerve probe and identify the nerve involved in the spasm then Dr. Choudhri would clip the nerve thus releasing the spasm. Melany wanted to try this because she desperately wanted relief.

I told the doctor a similar surgery had been suggested several years ago before the Buprenex had started relieving the spasms. We were concerned because they said she probably would lose a lot of her mobility and possibly not be able to sit up.

Dr. Rivener looked at Melany lying on the bed, all drawn up and hardly able to move. He looked at me and kindly asked, "And what can she do now?"

I had to admit, not much. We realized we had lived with Melany's gradually deteriorating condition so long we really did not see her as others did.

Dr. Rivener set up the surgery with Dr. Choudhri for the following Wednesday. They transported her back to St. Joseph and did all the necessary x-rays, tests and MRI.

We were all excited about the possibility of some of her pain being relieved. She was transferred back to MCG and the surgery was performed on June 28, 2005. Three doctors worked for twelve hours on her back. Dr. Rivever did his part and Dr. Kimberly Bingaman assisted Dr. Choudhri. Dr. Bingaman was expecting a baby and had several rest times. She reported to the full waiting room of our families and friends, many who stayed with us the entire time. She explained the procedure that the other doctors had told us they would do. She said they had performed a rhizotomy from T12 down to L4 in her spinal column. They actually removed part of her spine to get into the spinal column. She asked if Melany had ever had meningitis or any infection in her spine.

I told her that when Melany was twelve or thirteen she was in the hospital for twelve months and they had finally decided she had a contained virus in her spine. They treated her with massive doses of antibiotics and steroids. They did three myelograms and seven spinal taps during that year. She had lost her ability to walk and had to use a wheelchair.

I told her I did not know what a contained virus was. However, in later years when I told other medical professionals about that diagnosis they looked at me like I had three heads or something so I just forgot about it. Dr. Bingaman said that she knew what it was. She said it was an infection that apparently never completely cleared out and had crystallized in her spine. At some point it started breaking down in the spinal column and when she moved it was like grains of sand being rubbed against the sensitive part of her spine. She said it was a feeling similar to the sensation of sand being rubbed on a tender part of our body like the back of our hand.

The doctor asked how long had Melany complained with her back hurting. I told her I heard Melany tell someone not long ago she didn't remember not having a backache since she was thirteen. The doctor said they had scraped out something in her spinal column that looked like sand or small sea shells, and just removing those abrasive components should relieve a lot of her pain.

We asked why this had never been visible with all the tests that many good, caring physicians had ordered while trying to help her for these twenty-five years. Dr. Bingaman said the fact that the year she had all the spinal taps and myelograms they would have left a type of marker that would have prevented identifying anything else with other tests ordered or available.

We wept at the thought of all of those years of severe pain we had witnessed as the doctors had tried so hard to help her.

We were all excited with the anticipation of her being without at least some of the pain.

Everyone was so good to us at the MCG. Several of the nurses and the anesthesiologist at MCG Melany had known at St. Joseph for many years. The Neuro-Science Unit was fantastic. They allowed the family to stay in the end section of the large rooms in the Intensive Care Unit. They asked us to stay in our section when the doctors came in, and they would talk to us when they finished with Melany. This was a tremendous comfort to the patients and their families.

Melany had signed her DNR (do not resuscitate) papers and did not desire to be placed on a respirator. I asked her prior to her surgery to consider a respirator temporarily if she had pneumonia. She said only if it was something temporary that could be treated but only for a short time. She was agreeing only because she wanted to have a chance at a practically pain-free life.

On the third day after surgery Melany developed double pneumonia. She went into respiratory arrest and had to be put on a respirator. We were so thankful that she was alive and that she had agreed on the respirator earlier.

Many friends and family members came as they had done many times before. Church families everywhere were praying for her. As the days passed, I wondered what she meant by a "short time" on the respirator? I prayed I would know when the time was right that she had endured enough. Once again I had a peace that the Lord would let me know what to do and when to do it, because she was kept in a drug induced coma and could not respond.

After several attempts of trying to get her to breathe on her own, she was able to come off the respirator and was moved back to St. Joseph. Her lungs did not clear and she was getting progressively worse. Dr. Carmel Joseph was draining the fluid from her lungs when she had respiratory failure again. He was able to save her life again and she was placed on a respirator again for just a short time.

In a few weeks, Melany was able to go home. How happy everyone was, how very weak Melany still was. She had been through another difficult ordeal.

Melany's faith and peace prevailed that she was going to have a better life, with less pain in her back and nubs.

Once again we watched the wonderful prevailing peace in her life that was not affected by her circumstances or her situation.

As she trusted our loving, understanding Heavenly Father He granted to her all the peace that indeed passeth all human understanding."

"Blessed is he, who through long years of suffering,
Cut off from active toil,
Still shares by prayer and praise the work of others,
And thus devides the spoil."

"Blessed are thou, O child of God, who sufferest, and cannot
understand,
The reason for thy pain,
yet gladly leavest,
Thy life in His hand."

"Yea, blessed art thou whose faith is "not offended"
By trials unexplained by mysteries unsolved,
past understanding,
Until the goal is gained."
Freda Hanbury Allen

CHAPTER XII
<u>PEACE PERSEVERES</u>

*"I have learned whatever state I am in there
with to be content." Philippians 4:11*

Repeatedly while in the hospital, Melany had said that she had prayed that the Lord would allow her to return to St. Simons Island.

She had such wonderful memories of the good times that she had enjoyed through the years. When she was in college she would take her friends down to the beach. It was only an hour and forty-five minutes from her college. They had many fun-filled week-ends there. One week-end they had fifteen young people in a four room condo. What fun they had--what wonderful memories were made.

Through the years it had become increasingly difficult for her to ride. The last trip that she had made in the van had taken twelve hours, because the pain of motion was so great that we had to stop every few minutes. Usually the drive was four to five hours depending on the number of times that we had to stop with her. For several years we had to have her flown down in a private plane. It was so hard to get together all the supplies, equipment and things needed that we decided to stay for two months each year.

Melany thoroughly enjoyed our time there. She had a golf cart to ride on the beach, and collect seashells. Motorized vehicles (even golf carts) are not allowed on the beach but they had given her special permission to drive it there, because that was the only way that she could enjoy the beach. She also enjoyed fishing from the pier in the village. Very special to her was the fact that two of her former college friends lived on the island. One had two children and the other one had six. Melany enjoyed the children very much and really cherished the time that she spent with Julie and Noel and their families.

Since Melany had been unable to go for the previous two years, we had reserved the condo for November and December. She was very determined to go. The doctors knew that she was very weak but she gave them her old "clique," that she had used with family, friends and doctors for several years. She always said, "There are only two things that you need to remember. First and most importantly, when Jesus is ready for me, I am ready for him. Secondly, if I die on the way to St. Simons, while there or on the way home, you know that I died happy." They all agreed that they could not argue with that declaration.

Thus, we started making plans to go. We always take the majority of her supplies with us. The drill consisted of James taking a car load of supplies down, a friend pulls the golf cart and trailer with James' truck. He takes the extra oxygen concentrator, her electric wheel chair, the suction machine and a myriad of other things.

We knew this trip would be very challenging, because Melany was so ill. Her dad had moved the dining room table and had her hospital bed set up by the large double glass window. She could lie in bed and see the swimming pool below, and watch the children playing, as she had enjoyed doing so many times.

She could also the see the beach and the ocean and watch the boats and ships coming and going from the inter-coastal waterway. James had everything ready but it was a week before she was able to fly.

Melany always flies out one day, Jake usually flies with her. After I put her on the plane, I go home and reload the van and secure our houses to leave for two months. Then I would leave the next morning after getting a much needed overnight rest.

James picks her up at the airport on the island. They go to

the condo and order pizza, Melany usually sleeps until I get there the next morning.

Everything had been so different this time, as we prepared to leave. I wept privately as I packed her clothes. Melany had told me to only pack a few of her clothes and pack her a lot of long shirts and gowns because she knew that she was not going to be able to do the things that she usually did. She continued by saying that was alright, she would still be on the island and enjoy what she could. It still made me sad, realizing how much her condition had deteriorated since we had been to the beach two and a half years ago. It was very hard for James and I, knowing she would not be able to do many of the things that she had enjoyed so much before.

As I packed my things I had a very sad feeling again. I didn't pack my usual dress clothes, because I knew that I could not leave Melany to attend our church that we loved so much. I certainly would not be able to go out with the many friends that we had enjoyed through the years and had not seen for two years. But that too was alright with me. I had just asked God to please let us get her to St. Simons at least one more time, and grant her at least one more enjoyable Christmas on the island. We were close to getting the first prayer answered and I was very grateful!

When I took Melany to the airport, I was saddened again. Our dear long-time friends Charlie and Mary Joe Davis had flown Melany to the beach and back home for the last four years. What a blessing they had been through the years.

Charlie had been diagnosed with liver cancer just a few months before. He did not have a very good prognosis. However, he was there to fly with Greg Connell, who piloted the plane. He said that he just wanted to be there to help Melany if necessary. It really touched my heart to see Charlie fighting so valiantly to live and still being concerned about Melany. We are so blessed to have such wonderful friends.

I put Melany on the plane, watched it leave and said a

prayer for traveling mercies. Then I went home to finish packing.

As I drove the two hundred mile trip to the beach I thanked the Lord for all the good times that we had enjoyed there. I also thanked Him for giving me health and strength to be able to drive that distance. I wondered, at nearly seventy how many more times I would be alert enough to do this. I am always thankful for each day that God allows.

When Melany arrived at the beach, she had a great surprise. Her friends had gone over to the condo after James arrived and had decorated the condo with balloons and banners. The outside door was covered with pictures. The children had drawn pictures of Melany flying in an airplane and fishing and riding her golf cart on the beach.

Each year during November and December many of the homeowners come down. About ten of them had placed messages of welcome on the door as well. Her friends gave her the first night to rest after her flight. I came the next day and many friends visited that afternoon and night. It was exhausting for Melany, but lots of fun!

The beach experience was different. Jake had already been to the beach the week-end before and he was gone. James got us settled then he left for Vidalia, Georgia.

James had been working on an invention with a cousin in Vidalia for a little over a year. Vidalia is one hundred miles from Augusta and one hundred miles from St. Simons. He stayed in Vidalia during the week and came home every Thursday night and went back on Monday morning. He continued the same pattern while we were at the beach. Of course, he always came immediately if we needed him or when Melany was ill.

In August when we had felt that perhaps Melany would be able to go to the beach, we had to make a decision about what to do with Jake. Jake felt that he and his friend Bradley would be alright staying in Augusta while we were away.

They are very good responsible boys and are both very trust worthy. However, the thought of two seventeen year olds running a house alone for two months was a little unnerving.

Several friends in Augusta offered for Jake to stay with them, but two months with an extra teenager is a little much.

One of James' cousins came up with the perfect solution. Let Jake stay in the trailer with James in Vidalia and attend Robert Toombs Christian Academy in Lyons. It was a school similar to our church school, Curtis Baptist that he had attended all of his life. The two schools played each other in football and basketball.

Before we talked with Jake, we met with the school counselor and she worked with the counselor at the new school to coordinate all of his classes, so that he could go back to Curtis the second semester and graduate from there with his class. They worked it out beautifully.

When we told Jake, he resisted the idea, until we told him that he could play football and that RTCA had been state winners for two years. Then he was excited. Being a typical seventeen year old boy he was a little more interested in sports than academics.

So Jake had moved his clothes, TV and video games to Vidalia. He and his papa got along very well in the trailer. Jake also got to visit with a lot more cousins. I think James and Jake enjoyed not having the women-folk telling them what to do.

James came to the beach every week-end after Jake's football game and Jake came most of them. Occasionally he would go back to Augusta to visit with his friends. During the holidays, some of them came to the beach as well.

To add to the changes that we were experiencing, we had another sad thing to endure. When we had bought our condo, the first existing owners that we met had been Kevin and Bette McLoughlin. Although they resided in Mau Wau, New Jersey, they stayed on St. Simons for three to six months during the winter months each year to enjoy the nice weather that the south provided. We had enjoyed a very close relationship since that first meeting. They had moved into a lovely home on the island in 1997, the next year Kevin had been diagnosed with

Parkinson's Disease. Finally the diagnosis was changed to PSP (Progressive Supranuclear Palsy). He and Bette had endured some very difficult days for the last eight years. He had gone from being unsteady in walking to having real problems with his balance. Finally, losing his ability to speak. At this time he had started choking on his food, even though Bette would puree it. They had to insert a feeding tube to give him his needed nutrition. James and I had encouraged Bette and Kevin to come over and stay in their condo, so we could help Bette learn to care for Kevin's new feeding. I went up their condo three times a day until Bette felt confident in handling the new situation. Of course, as usual, she adapted quickly. They stayed on at the condo through Thanksgiving and Christmas, until we left in January. This trip was indeed quite different.

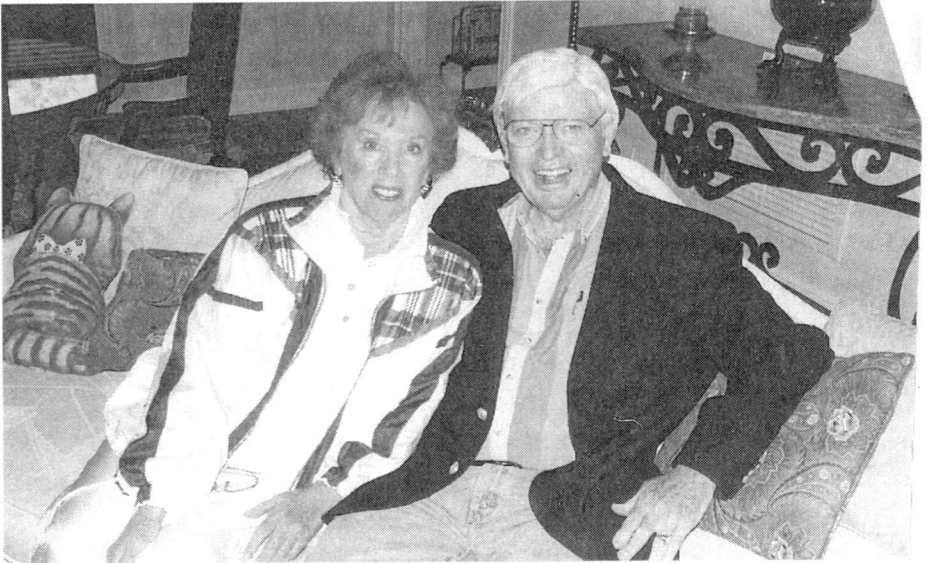

Bette & Kevin McLoughlin

Melany continued being very ill. Her heart rate went up to 230. Her oncologist sent us to a wonderful cardiologist. He did a lot of tests and concluded the same things that they had when she was twelve years old. The disease had either destroyed or imbalanced some sensor in her brain. While she was sitting still or even lying down the brain sensor sent the message that she was running uphill or exerting her body. Thus the heart would beat faster. It made her very, very weak and tired. After hospitalization, the doctor was finally able to get her heart rate down to 120.

We all felt so badly for Melany not being able to get out and go and do the few things that she enjoyed so much.

We had noticed a wonderful thing on this trip, however. After Melany had her back surgery in July we knew that she had almost no pain in her back compared to the many years of debilitating pain that she had endured. The plane ride down to the island and the return trip home was much more comfortable than ever before.

At the condo, she could ride her electric wheelchair down the long walkway from the elevator to the condo entrance without stopping several times. This was the first time ever that she could do this without severe pain. The movement of the chair bumping over the wooden planks had always made her pain almost unbearable. Now, she could just "zip" along.

As she expressed great joy over this great relief of her back pain, Melany had her calm attitude about not getting to do the enjoyable things. With her usual "make the best of any situation and enjoy what you can," she said, "Oh, well, there is always next year, and it will be better." We all prayed that it would be.

These verses described Melany attitude about life, at this time:

"As sorrowful, yet always rejoicing.
II Corinthians 6:10

Amid manifold trials, souls which love God will find reasons for bounding, leaping joy.
And it is possible in the darkest hour that ever swept a human life to bless the God and Father of our Lord Jesus Christ. Not simply to

endure God's will, nor only to choose it; but to rejoice in it with joy
unspeakable and full of glory.
<u>*STREAMS IN THE DESERT*</u>*-FROM TRIED AS BY FIRE*

Her deep abiding peace continued to persevere!

"O thou whose life of joy seems reft,
Of beauty shorn;
Whose aspirations lie in dust,
All bruised and torn,

Rejoice, tho each desire,
each dream,
Shall fall and fade,
It is the hand of love devine.

That holds the knife,
that cuts and breaks,
With tenderest touch,

That thou whose life
has borne some fruit,
May'st now bear much."
Annie Johnson Flint
STREAMS IN THE DESERT

CHAPTER XIII
<u>PERSEVERENCE PERSONIFIED</u>

"Blessed be God, even the Father of our Lord -- Jesus Christ,
the Father of mercies, and the God of all comfort.
Who comforted us in all our tribulation, that we may be able to
comfort them which are in any trouble,
By the comfort where with we ourselves are comforted of God."
II Corinthians 1:3&4.

After returning home in January 2006, our lives and routines continued as usual. For years, about the only thing different about us going on vacation was the changing scenery, because Melany's care and our responsibilities stayed the same. Changing scenery was nice though, and we were thankful for a change.

Melany continued getting weaker and it was becoming more difficult for her to breathe. In the early spring, I took her to her Pulmonary Specialist, Doctor Joseph. He did some breathing tests on her and made x-rays. As I was cleaning her oxygen machine a few days later, the phone rang. Because I had to finish and get her reconnected to the machine, I simply hit the speaker button on the phone. It was the nurse for the pulmonary doctor. She said that Dr. Joseph wanted me to bring Melany back the next day, and that he wanted me to have the rest of the family come as well. I explained that her father was out of town, but I would get in touch with him and we would all be there. When the call was completed, Melany said very matter-of-factly, "Mother, I guess you realize that when the doctor wants the entire family to come in that it is not good news." Of course, I was thinking the same thing.

I called her dad and he came home immediately. The next afternoon, Jake left school early and we all went to the doctor's office. Dr. Joseph is a wonderful, compassionate doctor. He showed us Melany's latest x-rays as he explained that the reason that she was having such difficulty breathing was because her diaphragm had almost stopped working. It was practically frozen in place and could no longer contract or expand. He said that the only thing that he could to do to help her was to place her on a respirator. He continued to explain that both a well known actor and a prolific singer had a type of artificial diaphragms that expanded with the help of a motor device, but Melany was not a candidate for one of those.

Melany said, "Dr. Joseph, you have a copy of my DNR. You know that in the derivative I state that I do not wish to be placed on a respirator ever again. So I will not do this. I'll just breathe as long as I can with oxygen, then I'll go to Heaven."

As the doctor stated the advantages of the newer machines, James and I just backed away. We had already promised, very painfully that we would see that her wishes were honored concerning this situation if she was unable to do so.

However, the doctor and Jake, both with tears in their eyes, continued encouraging her to try it. She refused, and finally said, "I'll tell you what doctor, you and Jake get hooked up to one for a week. If you both like it, I'll consider getting me one." They both agreed that they did not want to try it.

Very thoughtfully, Dr. Joseph said that a representative from a company that makes C-Pap breathing machines that people use for Sleep Apnea had been into his office that morning. He had demonstrated a machine called a Bi-Pap. The representative had left the information about the machine. The principle of the machine is that it helps to exchange the air in the lungs, not just force oxygen in. It was called a non-invasive respirator. He said that he should be able to get one in a couple of days, if she would try it. Melany agreed to try it.

The machine worked very well. It was a large piece of equipment that fit on the front platform of her wheel chair. The mask covered most of her small face, including her mouth and nose. It was similar to the mask of a pilot. This was a larger mask that she was not accustomed too. She would have to pull it away from her mouth to talk. But it did help her to breathe better. Everyone, including the doctor was very pleased.

Jake graduated from High School on the first of June. Melany was not able to attend. Jake went on to Georgia Southern University in the fall. He had planned in his mind and heart to go to "Mimi's School" since he was five years old. We were pleased with his choice.

Melany had already started planning for a trip to St. Simons Island in October. She was still very sick, but she could breathe much better, so she had great plans.

But when October came, Melany was in the hospital for most of the month, so she started planning for November. The first week of November, one of her favorite cousins died. She and Greg had always been very close, and they had gone to Georgia Southern together. She had led him into a real understanding of the assurance of his salvation. Later she had told him that she felt that the Lord would call him to be a preacher. He was quite shy, and declared to her that he could hardly speak up in his class, so there was no way in the world that he could ever preach but Greg continued growing closer to the Lord. Melany continued to pray that God would use him in a very special way. Eventually the Lord did call him into the ministry. He had studied hard, and had become the associate pastor of his church. We were all so proud of him. He had married a lovely girl, and she was a perfect pastor's wife.

Greg and Tressie had two beautiful children, Lindsey and Connor. Just when their life was going so well, Greg had been diagnosed with cancer. Of course Melany was extremely sad, as was all of the family and friends.

Several months later Greg went into the local hospice care

hospital. While there, he was a real inspiration to all that he came in contact with, as was his dear wife. James and Jake, who lived in Vidalia at the time, visited them often. Melany and Greg talked on the phone often even though they were both very weak, and at times could hardly hear each other. As Greg's condition worsened he became unable to talk most of the time, so they did not talk for a few weeks. As Tressie and I were talking on the phone one morning, Greg surprised us by asking to speak with Melany. Even though it was early in the morning, and she did not "do mornings," Melany was delighted. They teased each other often, she called him "Bub," and he called her "Sis." Tressie and I both had the phones on speaker. Although hardly audible, we heard Greg say, "Hey Sis. We have always been in competition. You always won academically, but I won in sports. Sis, I'm going to win this one. The doctor came in this morning and said that I might get to see Jesus before long. I'm going to win this one."

We were all crying as she replied, "Bub, don't count on it, it's still early and you haven't won yet. I may be there waiting on you." They both laughed. We all cried.

On November 3, 2006, the Lord mercifully called Greg Wiggins to his Heavenly home.

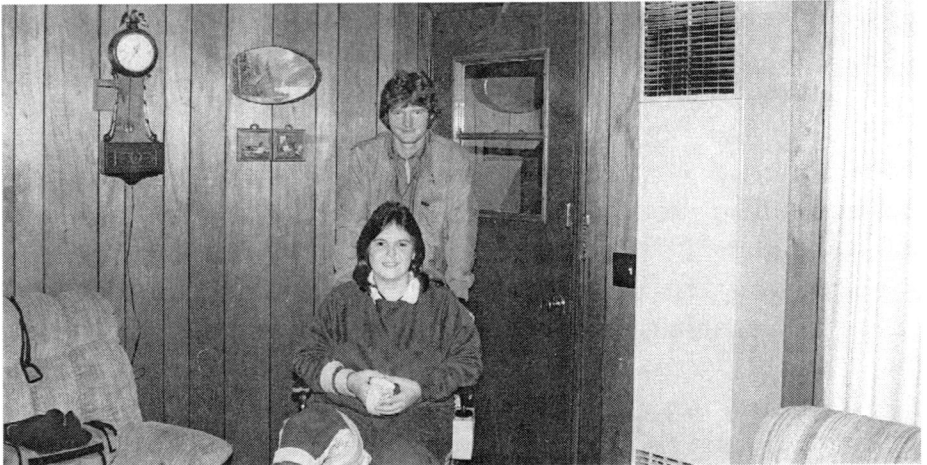

Melany & Greg

The second week in November we started the same drill of preparing her and her stuff for the beach. Charlie Davis, her pilot had died in the spring. A wonderful pilot, Steve Thompson had flown her down, because Greg Connell (Charlie's Co-Pilot) was unavailable. I was unable to follow as usual, because I had been sick when I had put her on the plane. Julie came to the condo and helped James with Melany's needs until I could go. After I arrived at the beach and went to the doctor, I was diagnosed with Congestive Heart Failure. We knew that this stay was probably going to be more difficult than last year. However we were all accustomed to changes in plans and trying to enjoy whatever we could.

Melany's Bi-Pap Machine was working well, and she had great expectations of being able to do some of the things that she had been unable to do the year before. Although we knew that she was not any better physically, she could breathe better, and we all had high hopes for her and her desires.

We knew that Melany's condition had deteriorated since last year. She only weighed sixty-five pounds. But for us, it had been gradual. As friends came to visit, they were shocked by her appearance. One of our friends walked in the door and turned and walked out without a word. His wife went out to see what was wrong. He was standing on the walk-way weeping. It was also quite unnerving for her school mates to see her as she was now. However, they continued to come and add joy to her life even though for the most part she was still not able to go anywhere or do anything.

Melany's normal week at the beach is as follows:

She will spend one day at the beach on her golf-cart shelling. She points out where the shells or the mounds are, and depending on who her "Shell-dog" is, they pick them up for her. Even one of her doctors that lives down the beach from us would often come and go with her. Melany enjoyed these excursions immensely. She could out-last all of us, of course she was riding and we were walking or riding and climbing on and off of the cart.

She will rest the next day and then the next day she will go fishing. Fishing has been a passion for her since she was a little girl.

She rests another day, then the next afternoon she and Julie go to the pier and watch the most gorgeous sunsets imaginable. They will usually hang out at the pier (often other friends join them) and watch the night fishermen catching fish, crabs and sharks. Melany enjoys all of these activities.

Melany goes once a week to the Oncologist to get her port-a-cath needle changed and to get fluids. Occasionally, we have to take her to the Cardiologist or the emergency room.

Basically, if we are there sixty days, she shells sixteen times, goes fishing sixteen times and goes to the pier sixteen times. Then she goes to the doctor at least eight times.

This last trip of ninety days, she shelled ten times, fished eight times and went to the pier fifteen times. She went to the doctors or hospital fifteen times. I went once or twice weekly.

When one of her doctors came to see us and expressed that he and his wife missed seeing her on the beach and that they were so sorry that she could not do the things that she usually did. Melany had her usual "make the best of any situation and enjoy what you can" attitude. She said, "Well, if I've got to be in the bed most of the time, there is no better scenery anywhere than here!"

We had our last Thanksgiving and Christmas at St. Simons. Somehow I believe that we all realized that it might be our last one there. We were not able to attend the usual festivities or worship services. Especially the very special Christmas Eve Service that we had always attended at First Baptist (our church on the island). One year Melany had pneumonia (of course we didn't realize it at the time), she insisted on going to the Christmas Eve Service, we had to take her to the ER as soon as we left the church.

We missed attending the "Messiah" at the Methodist Church. We were unable to go out with our friends, attend the many parties and "get-to-gathers" that we were a part of during the holidays. Nor did we do any entertaining, although many of our friends came and visited.

However, we had a very nice Thanksgiving and Christmas, surrounded by many caring friends.

While we were rather house confined, Melany and I began to write this book. I had been encouraged by several friends, Joyce, June, Pat, Nelda and Margaret to write a book about Melany's early escapades.

Then her teachers, (who knew her well), Bobbie Moyer (Playschool), Bobbie McKnight (Kindergarten). as well as Rene Shoemaker and Gerry Holt (two of her early Grade School Teachers) insisted that I should indeed share her early life and of her determination to survive and enjoy life after she became sick. Also, how she was such a fine student and developed into such a fine and gracious young lady.

James and Jake were gone most of the week, so we would write and then share the manuscript with them when they came for the week-ends. We had much enjoyment and fun writing the first chapters entitled Prittle and Prattle.

However, the chapters on Pain and the rest of the book through Peace were more difficult. We laughed and we cried as we wrote. It was quite an adventure.

I was glad that we could write it together, because we could help each other remember the journey. Melany wanted very much for the book to help others. She had the same positive attitude that she had always displayed and her faith had always revealed. Melany's desire was for this book:

FIRST, to glorify God, His love, faithfulness and sustaining grace.

SECOND, to thank and honor the medical professionals and all the many doctors for their dedication and hard work for all the many years that they tried so faithfully to help her.

THIRD, to express her heartfelt gratitude to our church staff and members for their visits, cards and prayers.

FOURTH, to thank the many loving family members and friends for their prayers, and the many days and hours they spent caring for all of us.

WE WILL ALWAYS REMEMBER:
The PRITTLE --
And the many delightful and enjoyable days!
The PRATTLE --
With all the fun we had!
The PAIN --
Covered by God's sustaining grace and the   comfort that He provided.
The PRAYER --
The most wonderful gift that God has given to us other than our salvation.
        The strength experienced when we prayed.
            The support when others prayed for us.
The sustaining grace that keeps us near to the heart of God.
The PRAISE --
The key that truly unlocks the door to answered
Prayer and many blessings.

The PEACE --
The wonderful feeling within our heart and soul
and spirit that is not affected by circumstances or situations.
            TO GOD BE THE GLORY!!

* * * * *

Now, I must complete the book with the last chapters. From the time in December 2006 when Melany and I finished what we thought would complete the book until February 2008, when God in His love and care called my dear husband and soulmate James to his Heavenly home.

Three months later in May, He reached down in His great love and tender mercy, and relieved Melany of her many years of pain and suffering and took her to her perfect peace and rest.

It will be an arduous task to describe the brave way that they both faced their final days and left this world for their Heavenly Home and their rewards.

I have now buried all four of my children, and my dear husband. God has always been faithful to me and I will seek to be faithful to Him in seeking to finish the last part of this book.

My earnest prayer is that it will:
    praise,
        honor,
            glorify
                and please the Lord!

Out of suffering have emerged the strongest souls; the most massive characters are seamed with scars; martyrs have put on their coronation robes glittering with fire, and through their tears have the sorrowful first seen the gates of Heaven.
Chapin

"We shall know by the gleam and glitter
Of the golden chain you wear,
By your heart's calm strength in loving,
Of the fire you have had to bear.

Beat on, true heart, forever;
Shine bright, strong golden chain;
And bless the cleansing fire and
The furnace of living pain!"
Adelaide Proctor
STREAMS IN THE DESERT

CHAPTER XIV
<u>PERFECTION</u>

"A good man showeth favor, and lendeth; he will guide his
affairs with discretion."
Psalm 112:5.

When we returned home in late January 2007, I had finished a bout with congestive heart failure. I had begun my fourth battle against cancer, which by the grace of God is now in remission.

Jake was back at college in Statesboro and James was in Vidalia working with his cousin J.R. on the invention. February was very difficult for Melany. She was back in the hospital for six weeks. Friends continued calling, sending notes and cards of encouragement and visiting her when she was able for visits.

The end of June one of the many younger cousins graduated from high school. Jake and James went down to Vidalia for a family graduation party the day before the graduation. The "younger friends" party was held after the graduation ceremony.

They stayed in a motel and James became very ill with severe nausea and was unable to attend the party. He was sick all night and the next day he was still sick and unable to attend the graduation. He insisted that Jake go on and go the party afterward. The next day Jake called me (we had talked several times since their arrival), and he said, "This is not just a virus, something is bad wrong with Papa." Jake had given him lots of fluids as had the older cousins that had come over to check on him. Jake had tried to get him to go to the Emergency Room. He refused, even with the prodding of the other family members.

Jake needed to leave and go to Statesboro to clean out his

apartment. Of course I couldn't leave Melany and go down, and I knew his family could and would take good care of him.

Jake had called two of James cousins, J.R. and Walter. They couldn't talk him into going to the ER, because he said he would be alright. He didn't want to go home with either of them, because he didn't want to expose either family to his virus. J.R. called his wife (James' first cousin), Katherine and she came and insisted (she can be very persuasive) that James would go home with them. James was too weak to object, so he went. They took very good care of him until he came home the next week-end, still not feeling well.

The first week-end in July was the Powell reunion, so James stayed in Vidalia for that, and Jake joined him. The second week-end James came home very hoarse. The third week-end he had laryngitis and could hardly whisper. After much begging from me he agreed to stay home on Monday and go to the doctor. He reasoned before, that he and J.R. would sit out under the large oak trees, get real hot and then go in to the air conditioned house or office, so that was causing the hoarseness and he would be alright soon. Anyway, he added, he was coming home on Wednesday to celebrate our anniversary.

On Monday our pulmonary doctor (Carmel Joseph) x-rayed him and did some other tests. He sent him to an ENT doctor who said that he could not say why, but James' vocal chords were frozen. He felt that he could do a procedure and try to correct the situation. On Tuesday evening, Dr. Joseph called and wanted me and James to come in on Wednesday morning.

We listened in stunned disbelief as he gently told us that James had a tumor one-half the size of his left lung. It had apparently burst out of the lung and somehow the lung had resealed itself. Thus, he was not short of breath, nor did he cough. He felt that it had happened the last of June, when he was so sick and throwing up blood.

Dr. Joseph was almost certain that it was malignant so he set us up to go to Dr. Hudson, my and Melany's Oncologist on

Friday. The x-rays revealed that the growth was wrapped around the vocal cord, causing the laryngitis. It was also wrapped around the Aorta and lying on the heart. So he said of course it was inoperable. We already had reservations for the night at a hotel near our home (we could not go far from Melany). We always did this on our anniversary.

One of Melany's nurses and a friend stayed with her. Of course we were two miles away and Jake was right next door and checked on them often.

I already had our overnight bags packed, so we went home to get them and to give the caretakers further instructions via my numerous lists. We did not tell anyone our devastating news.

We went on to the hotel still in shock and disbelief. We had a good cry in our room and went down for a romantic candlelight dinner. We had an unusually precious and special fifty-second anniversary celebration. We went home on Thursday afternoon. We had decided to wait until we went to Dr. Hudson on Friday before we told anyone. It was hard to act as if everything was alright when it really wasn't and probably never would be. I remember that my eyes literally burned as I fought to hold back the tears.

We went to the oncologist and he ordered more tests. James had to be admitted to the hospital and have the thoracic surgeon that had performed his heart by-pass, Dr. Catalino, to open up his chest and do a biopsy to determine what type of cancer he had. It was determined to be squamous cell carcinoma-- inoperable and incurable. They told me that he could live two to three years with radiation and chemotherapy.

We went to our friend Dr. Byron Dasher, Radiologist. The doctors all worked together and decided that Dr. Dasher would administer the radiation treatments and then Dr. Hudson would do the chemotherapy. Our hearts were so heavy as the situation moved so rapidly.

James went for his last dove shoot on opening day of the season, the Saturday before Labor Day. On Labor Day he and

Jake went with friends to our annual Labor Day barbecue at the lake. The guys always went to a dove shoot in the afternoon. But James chose to come home so we could go back to the hotel for the afternoon, evening and night. We had the usual caretakers for Melany. I teased him and told him that I knew he must really love me to give up a dove shoot. He was to start radiation on Tuesday morning and we somehow knew some things would never be the same again. We savored that really memorable time.

James did well with the radiation. He was able to go back to Vidalia several times. Then in late October he started the chemotherapy treatments.

Melany was getting weaker and so was James. Our friends all stayed strong and very caring and encouraging to us.

The week before Thanksgiving Jake drove James to Vidalia and then to Pooler, Ga. Where my nephew, Lamar had just opened a satellite office from our Canada office. It was the last trip that James was able to make. James' condition started deteriorating rapidly.

The care of James and Melany had become very physically difficult. I could not have made it if the family had not come and helped me several times a week. I was very grateful that James had eighty-nine first cousins still living (he had ninety-nine). They came from many miles away to help out. His Daddy was one of twelve and his Mother had fourteen brothers and sisters. We have always been close to all of them. I do not have a lot of family left, and none of them live near. I have always loved all of James' family dearly, they endeared themselves even more to me daily with their help and care. My Sunday School Class and many other friends set up a schedule and brought food almost daily. We received many cards and letters of encouragement.

Melany had found a poem and printed it out. I put it in a frame and hung it in view of James' recliner. I placed another by the bed. It said:

WHAT CANCER CANNOT DO
**Cancer is so limited..
It cannot cripple love,
It cannot shatter hope,
It cannot eat away at peace,
It cannot destroy confidence,
It cannot kill friendship,
It cannot shut out memories,
It cannot silence courage,
It cannot invade the soul,
It cannot reduce eternal life,
It cannot quench the spirit,
It cannot lessen the power
Of the Resurrection.**-Author Unknown

*"In all things we have complete victory through Him
who loved us!...There is nothing in all creation that
will ever be able to separate us from the love of God which is ours
through Christ Jesus our Lord."*   Romans 8:37-39

On December 5, 2007, the test that they did on James showed that the tumor had shrunk fifty per cent. We were all ecstatic!

James wanted to buy special Christmas presents for me, Melany & Jake. He had Jake take him shopping, very unusual for him, he did not like to shop. I received a beautiful watch. They took Melany and let her pick out her own watch (she wanted one with a large face, with date, etc. on it). Jake picked out a nice computer.

On Christmas Eve our grandaughter Frannie, came with her husband Jeremy and two year old Isaiah. Many friends and family members visited. We all enjoyed having a two year old's excitement on Christmas morning.

As busy as things were, I wanted to cook for Christmas Eve and Christmas Day. I made sure that I fixed everything I knew that James enjoyed. I believe that I knew in my heart that this might be the last Christmas Dinner that we would share. He did not have very much taste now, and he would often choke and sometimes have to be suctioned.

We embraced the wonderful Holiday Season and I tried to make it as normal as it could be.

Even as his weight constantly dropped, he was unable to eat much and became weaker day by day, James attitude stayed positive. He was often in pain yet he continued to be kind and loving to all. He was so dear to me! One day I was in the utility room washing clothes, James came in, embraced me and gave me a poem that he had torn out of a book. James was not a poetry lover so it meant a lot to me for him to select it.

The poem is as follows:

"When I Must Leave You"
When I must leave you for a little while,
Please do not grieve and shed wild tears;
And hug your sorrow to you through the years;
But start out bravely with a gallant smile;
And for my sake and in my name,
Live on and do all things the same.
Feed not your loneliness on empty days,
But fill each waking hour in useful ways.
Reach out your hand in comfort and in cheer,
And I in turn will comfort you and hold you near;
And never, never be afraid to die,
For I am waiting for you in the sky!
Helen Steiner Rice

In the beginning of his illness, James claimed part of II Kings 20:2-6a. *When Hezekiah was sick unto death verse 2 says, "Then he turned his face to the wall, and prayed unto the Lord saying, (3) I beseech thee, O Lord, remember now how I have walked before thee in truth and with a perfect heart and have done that which is good in Thy sight. And Hezekiah wept sore."*

God told Isaiah (the prophet) to tell Hezekiah (5b)"*I have heard thy prayer, I have seen thy tears; behold I will heal thee.*" *(6a) "And I will add unto thy days fifteen years.*"

This was what we prayed and believed for. James said that he wasn't asking God for fifteen years, only enough time to set his affairs in order, physically, financially and spiritually, and to let his family and friends know how much he loved and appreciated them. He was certainly able to do that. He never asked me or the doctors how much time that they thought he might have.

Early on, James had told us, and his doctors as well as the many pastors, family and friends. "I am completely committed to God and I have committed my loved ones to His care. The Lord can heal me here, or in Glory, it's up to Him."

God chose Glory with all of its wonderful pain free splendor.

Our family members and friends were so precious. As I had mentioned earlier, some came from out of town every week to help me with James and Melany.

When Jake came home for the Thanksgiving Holidays, it was a short time, during which he took James on his last trip. Many friends visited and we were very thankful for all of our blessings.

It was only a week until Jake came home for the Christmas season which was very busy. Jake realized what a difficult time I had caring for James and Melany. They were both so ill by then, that I was trying to stay between both condos during the night. I would stay with James in the evenings (when we did a lot of sharing), married couples can have a lot of nurturing intimacy that is very dear. James and I would have our evening devotions and James would go to sleep after the eleven o'clock news.

By that time Melany was finished with her evening television programs. I would do the things that I had to do to get her and her equipment ready for the night. She always stayed up late, so I would go back over to our condo, check on James and set the clock for one hour. Then, I would go back to sleep for an hour with Melany. Set the clock for another hour and go sleep with James for an hour. I had continued to do this every night since the beginning of November, except the week-ends and during the holidays when Jake would sleep over with his Papa. Then I would just sleep at Melany's. I was close to exhaustion, but God was faithful to sustain me.

Jake went back to college in January and returned home three days later. He had taken his exams and unenrolled himself for the semester. He said, "Nana, I didn't know until I was home for Christmas what a hard time you were having. I just couldn't leave you to do all of this alone."

What a wonderful grandson God had blessed us with. I was sorry that he was out of college, but so very glad to have him home to help. I don't know what I would have done for the next few difficult months without him.

January was physically and emotionally hard for all of us. Melany seemed to be getting a little stronger. James was getting weaker. Most of the time he had to be held by his arms and walked to the bathroom, chair or bed.

For many years Melany's friends came to celebrate her birthday. So on Wednesday night, January 30, 2008, the "gang" gathered. This time they brought the cake, ice cream and all the goodies.

That day James had felt a little stronger. He wanted to attend a Retirement Luncheon for a friend. His good friend, Al Rodgers and Jake took him. They both came home quite distressed. James had lost a hundred and forty pounds in three months. They said that friends would walk by and not recognize him. He couldn't speak, so Al would call them over. He said that it was hard to see the shock on their faces.

James had rested after he had returned from his difficult time attending the luncheon. He wanted to come over to Melany's to see her and her friends. Jake brought him over for a few minutes.

After giving Melany a beautiful birthstone ring with

diamonds, her Dad kissed her for the last time. Jake walked him back across the patio to our condo. I went with them to help get James ready for bed. When I returned to Melany's, two of her friends said after her Dad left crying, she cried (very unusual for her), and said, "I will never see my Dad alive again." And she didn't.

Thursday and Friday was very hard, James was very weak and short of breath. Both days he wanted us to help him out on our back patio, for us to sit by the lake. We had spent many happy hours there in the past, and had many thoughtful discussions during the last few months. We sat in the warm sunshine, held hands and kissed and said many meaningful things to each other.

Saturday was horrendous. James was literally smothering and gasping for breath. He refused to let me call the doctor, or go to the hospital. He wanted to stay at home. Several friends were there most of the day.

Al and Don Leverette came, and we took him inside. He sat in his recliner. He would extend his hand and arm upward, and utter some words that we couldn't hear. Finally Jake asked him what he was doing. He whispered, "Just reaching for Jesus, and telling Him I am ready." Al and Don would not leave us. They begged him to go to the hospital. I wanted very badly for him to go, but he had said many times (just as Melany said), that he wanted to die at home. We just couldn't believe that the end was near.

One of our doctors had told me in early January that he felt I should know that he did not think James could last until summer. I hadn't listened. I have stated, James had never asked me or any of the doctors what time line they thought he had.

By night, James was resting and breathing easier, after he went to sleep, Jake told me to go and stay with Melany. His friend Nate Tanner was going to spend the night with him to help him with James, if needed. They promised me that they would call me if he woke up.

Two friends had stayed with Melany all day, so I went over

so they could leave. We talked for a while, and she told me, "Daddy is very tired, we are going to have to let him go. You know that he is not going to get any better, only worse." I did not voice it to her, but I thought of all the times that doctors, friends and family had said that to me about her. I just couldn't let them go. I could not imagine life without either one of them.

I was so tired, I finished getting Melany ready for the night and I went to sleep about two o'clock. Jake called at five, he had gotten up to check on James and found him of the floor, at the foot of the bed. He was wedged between the bed and the dresser. Jake and Nate had tried to get him up, and they couldn't. He was so frail that they were afraid that they would break his bones trying to lift him, so they had called the ambulance. Jake rode in the ambulance with James, and Nate followed them. I called June, our friend of fifty years, who was now our neighbor. She came right down to stay with Melany and I drove the mile and a half to the hospital.

Dr. Joseph was out of town, so Dr. Behnia came to the hospital. He ordered x-rays and fluids. The x-rays revealed that James had pneumonia in both lungs. Dr. Behnia immediately started intravenous antibiotics. He said that James was very ill, and that Dr. Joseph would be back Monday morning, and would do a bronchoscopy (Kinda like a bronchial rotor-rooter), which would remove the mucus and help him to breathe better. But he wanted to get the medicines in him first.

Joyce and Roy came immediately. Roy went on to church, and Joyce stayed with me, as she always had done through the years. After church many friends came. James was in the emergency room until that evening at five o'clock, because they did not have a room available.

Although he was weak, he was laughing and talking. I was much encouraged and really thought that after the procedure the following morning, he would get to go home and be better for a while.

James had been too sick to eat lunch, but by dinner time he

was much improved and hungry. They brought him his tray of jello, soup, pudding and tea. He jokingly said, "I hope this is not my last meal, I would prefer a big juicy steak." We all laughed. I assured him that he would have one as soon as he could go home. Joye Neal was coming at five o'clock so Joyce could go home with Roy. I went home to check on Melany and to tell her that her Daddy was feeling much better, and would probably be home by Tuesday.

Before she left, Joyce fed her dear friend of over fifty years, his last meal (maybe he had a steak in Heaven). In the note that I wrote to Joyce and Roy, I thanked them for always being there for us in an emergency, or just a time of need. I also expressed to Joyce that I could not think of anyone that James had rather have to feed him his last meal on earth than her. They had always shared a good time of fun and laughter.

Joye's name fits her happy, exuberant personality. She and James also shared fun times. When I returned she had James laughing and she said she had sung to him, and he had tried to sing with her.

Joye said that James had asked her to call me and see when I was coming back, because he wanted her to be able to leave before dark because she doesn't see well to drive after dark. As she related this to me, she had tears in her eyes. She said that as sick as he was, he was still concerned about others. He always was.

James was very tired and in great pain, after lying on a small bed with a thin pad in the ER all day. They had to put him in a room with another man. The man had a lot of noisy company, and although he loved people, the activity and noise was really getting to James. I asked the nurse to call the doctor and see if they could move him, possibly to the Intensive Care unit. She said that he was not sick enough for that.

Jake had been back and forth between the hospital and checking on Melany and taking a nap. He was going to stay with James for the night, because they wouldn't let me stay since he shared a room with a gentleman. This was the night of the super bowl. I told him to go on home, because his friends had planned to come over to watch the game at our place (James had looked forward to this as well). Then when it was over, he could come back to the hospital and stay with James for the night, and I would go home, and stay with Melany. Also during the game he would be next door to Melany's if they needed anything there.

James did not want to watch the Super Bowl, he just wanted to talk. James and I had a loving time. I climbed up on his bed, amid all the tubes (they were on one side), and we snuggled. We talked about how much better he was feeling and knowing that he would be better to-morrow after the cleaning procedure.

When Jake came back to the hospital around eleven thirty, I was sitting close to James' bed. He started telling me again, in just a whisper how much he loved me and the children. He motioned for Jake to come close to the other side of the bed.

He continued as he said to me, "I fell in love with you the first time I saw you. I have never desired another woman. You have always fulfilled all my needs and taken excellent care of me, our children and both of our families, and many others. You have never disappointed me in anyway. I've always loved and adored you, and I still do." He told Jake that when he chose a wife, to look for one just like his Nana.

Jake had heard enough, (I really don't think that he wants a wife like his grandmother) he walked outside. Then I repeated some of our earlier sharing and told him how much I had always loved him and still did. Again, I thanked him for always taking such good care of me, our children, his family and mine. Also what strength he had given to me and what a wonderful example he had been to our children and grandchildren.

He asked me to sing one of our favorite songs, that we often sang to each other. It was hard, but I did it somehow. After I tearfully sang "You Are my Sunshine, my only sunshine, you make me happy when skies are gray. You'll never know dear how much I love you, please don't take my sunshine away." Then he asked me to sing "Amazing Grace." I made it through the first stanza, and he wanted me to sing the last one. He tried to sing with me, "When we've been there ten thousand years, bright shining as the sun. We've no less days to sing His praise than when we first begun."

Jake had come back in. I knew that I had to get out of there quickly or I was going to fall completely to pieces. I told James (I always called him sweet and he called me little sweet), that Jake was staying with him for the night and I was going home to care for Melany.

As I kissed him, he grabbed my arm and said, "Please take me home with you." I assured him that I would be back early to-morrow morning before Dr. Joseph took him to the procedure room. We would go home as soon as Dr. Joseph would let us.

I left and Jake stayed. He had to try to sleep in a straight-backed chair, because the room was so small. I felt badly for him and I told him so. He insisted he wanted to stay. I repeat: what a great grandson!

As I went to my van, I sang in my head and heart, "Lord, please don't take my sunshine away." Never thinking that my sunshine was almost gone and I would never again see his smiling face. I've wished many times that I had not left him.

I drove the two miles home. June went home. I had taken my shoes off and got Melany and me something to drink. I was telling her that her Dad was better. The phone rang and I said that was probably Jake calling to say her Dad was already asleep.

Very excitedly Jake said, "Nana, come quick, Papa's heart has stopped. They are in the room now with the paddles to shock him back." James always slept on his right side, however Jake said that he had turned over on his left side, gave a little sigh and stopped breathing. Jake said that he ran out and got help, they called a code and immediately the room filled with helpers. He was quite shaken.

I told him to go in and tell them that the paddles were OK, but nothing more, because he had signed a DNR. I told him I would be there shortly.

I will never forget the look of pain and despair on Melany's face, when I told her what Jake had said. Our world was crashing, and we couldn't stop it.

I called my neighbor to come stay with Melany and I was at the hospital in five minutes. Jake met me at the entrance to the hospital. He said, "Nana, he is really gone!" We went up the room, I was praying all the way that it really wasn't true. That somehow they had been able to bring him back. Of course, he was gone. Jake reiterated what had happened and he left to go stay with Melany so Elizabeth could go back to her family.

The doctor came in and the nurse asked if he was an organ donor. They said that because of the chemotherapy nothing could be used except his eyes. They called the eye bank. Someone from the eye bank then called me and said someone would be there as soon as possible. The nurse said that I could sign some papers when they came, and then leave. She said that I stay as long as I wanted to.

I sat by James' bed in disbelief and horror. I kissed him, hugged him. I poured my heart out to him, our entire life together for fifty three years (actually with our engagement it was fifty four). Fifty four wonderful years was over in one heart beat. I told him over and over how much I had always loved and appreciated him. I repeated much of what I had said just one hour or so ago, before I had left the hospital.

Around three am a nurse came in and said they could not use his eyes because he had tested for some kind of eye disease. She asked if she could call the funeral home. I said OK, I was going to stay until they came to get his body.

She said that she had been there when they first came in and they had felt a very faint heartbeat in his neck. She went on to say that if they had not been told to stop the paddles they could have possibly brought him back.

This broke my heart because I felt that I had stopped the code. As I was writing this chapter and weeping I asked Jake to help me with the accuracy of that painful night. I shared with him what the nurse had said to me and I expressed the extreme heartache that I had because I had been responsible for stopping the code.

Jake said, "No, Nana I didn't tell them a thing you said. When I got back to the door of the room, they were all coming out. Apparently, they had realized that he had a DNR." He said, "I think I told you this before." He may have, but I did not hear it or I would not have been so regretful for three years.

I am so grateful to know this now. I did not feel guilt for these three years, but extreme sadness and sorrow, thinking I might have been responsible for cutting his life short.

I did remember that the day after James died Dr. Joseph had called, I did not tell him what the nurse had said, but I asked did he think they could have brought him back if they had not stopped the code. He kindly said, "Back to what? To go through this again and perhaps again?"

I replied, "No, he was ready to die. I just wasn't ready." A reality I have faced many times since then.

When the funeral director came, it was an old friend of James' that he had served with in service forty six years ago. I drove home alone, still feeling numb and dazed, continuing to pray that this was just a dream and I would surely wake up.

Jake was with Melany, so we all talked for a long time, until almost daylight. I shared with them some of the precious things that he had said to me. They each had thoughts of their own to share.

I was exhausted but I only slept two hours, because I always had to start early taking care of Melany and her needs.

Jake called Joyce and Roy, and they came. I called James' cousin Roger (he was like a brother to James) and his wife Rosa. They came immediately from their home eighty miles away. They were always available to help.

When they arrived, we called other family members and went to the funeral home to start plans for the funeral and burial.

Later that afternoon, I had to take Melany down to St. Josephs Hospital to have her huber needle changed. Her van, which was the only vehicle we had that could handle two wheelchairs had been stalling occasionally. The mechanic had not been able to find the cause nor a solution for it. Roger and Rosa were following us in their car, in case we had trouble. The van cut off four times in the five mile trip.

When we got to the hospital, I called the disabled van company that serviced the lift and hand controls on our van. They rent vans that are handicapped equipped, with lifts. They were closing, but they kindly waited for us to get there. I rented that van for a month, before purchasing a new one.

*   *   *   *   *

Our church did not have a minister at this time. I called our former minister and friend, Mark Harris who was now serving a church in Charlotte, N.C.   He could not come for the service until Friday.

We had visitation at the funeral home on Wednesday and Thursday nights. We chose two nights because when Ric died, we were so overwhelmed by the number of people that came. We had planned his visitation from seven to nine. At ten-thirty there were still people waiting in line to speak to us. It was eleven before everyone left. We knew that our friends were much older now, so we felt that this was better for all. Melany was able to go to the funeral home for a couple of hours, she enjoyed seeing the many friends that she had not seen for years.

So many friends came, men that had worked with James, family, church family and neighbors. Many of them shared memories and stories with us.

James was a job steward for many years at SRS and Plant Vogtle. Ordinarily, the Job Steward is not a favorite person, because they are the liaisons between the workers, contractors and the unions. It is often a difficult position. Many men said that James was the kindest most helpful person that they had ever known. As the men discussed this with us, they all agreed that he could get the job done.

Three of the younger men who had worked together said that James had called them into his office one day for a talk. They said he had smiled, was pleasant and encouraging as usual. He told them that they must have a lot of stress, turmoil and probably unhappiness in their lives for them to display such anger and impulsive behavior at work. He said, "Let's pray about it." They said that they were shocked, but appreciative of him caring for them.

When they left, they said they looked at each other and remarked that we realized that we had just been reprimanded, corrected and disciplined without a harsh word. But, they continued we got the message that he would not tolerate our current attitudes anymore.

He could correct our children the same way. However, he could get a little sterner and louder with repeated offenses.

Four people came that he had given cars to and they expressed gratitude for his thoughtfulness. Others told of borrowed money that he would not accept payment for if he thought they couldn't afford it.

Two sisters came who were our neighbors when they were young teenagers. One lived in a town about thirty miles from here, and the other one lived hundreds of miles away and was visiting her sister. I was so glad to see them and so was Melany and Jake. Jake especially enjoyed the stories that they told him about his Daddy as they were growing up together.

They reminded me of one Christmas Eve, many years ago. All of our family was gathered at our house for Christmas Eve. Melany had not been able to go to the aunt's house, so the family all came to ours.

The girls' parents were good parents but sometimes were heavy drinkers (especially the mom). They came often to our house for a "little break." This night, their parents were intoxicated and verbally fighting. They were frightened, so they came to our house. Realizing that we were having a family celebration, they started to leave. James insisted that they stay.

After our dinner, we always saved desert until after the gifts were exchanged, we all gathered in our large den and James read the Christmas Story with the help of Melany and two young cousins. Then he prayed, thanking God for all of our blessings, for our wonderful family, and for the two girls, calling them by name and thanking God for their parents and asking God to bless them, bring them closer to him and bless their entire family. He then reminded God that we had prayed for this family many times before.

The adults exchanged gifts on Christmas Eve, and we all gave gifts to the children. We gave small token gifts (clothes, pajamas, boots, etc. and one toy) to our children. Then the children received their long desired gifts on Christmas Morning. While the others were eating dinner, I had quickly taken the names off of gifts we had for some family members (I told them what I was doing), and friends that we would not see until after Christmas. I put the girls names on the gifts so that when we exchanged gifts they each had several. They were much appreciative.

Then James went to their house, and asked the couple if their daughters could spend the night, because they were having such a good time with all the children. He had no word of rebuke for them. The parents agreed and things were better the next day. The parents called early, they were going to mass and were going out for a family Christmas dinner.

The girls told me they realized that we were probably the only neighbors that really seemed to like their parents, and truly cared for them. They also said that was the first time that they remembered hearing their names called in prayer.

The girls said they had decided then, at a young age that they wanted a loving family like we had and wanted to always celebrate Christmas Eve and Christmas Day as we did. What a heart-rending compliment for a family that certainly was far from perfect. But we did always express love!

A young man in his forties came. I had known that James had hunted with his father and him (when he was young). His father had worked with James one time. The man told us that James was always so good to his family. His mother had left the family when he was thirteen. His dad had become very depressed and started drinking heavily. He was no longer dependable to him or his grandparents who lived next door in a trailer.

He said his dad would always stay sober when he knew Mr. Wiggins was coming to hunt. He said he always chose to walk with James instead of his dad. James always brought a gun for him and for his dad to use, because Dad had pawned or sold their guns.

He said the Christmas that he was fifteen was bleak financially and gift wise. He went on to say on Christmas morning his dad was drunk so he went up to his grandparents. His grandmother was fixing a wonderful Christmas dinner complete with turkey and all the trimmings.

He asked where all the food came from. His grandfather said Santa came last night, He brought lots of food and he left something under the tree for you. There he found a long box with a new shotgun just like the one that James had. There was a metal plate on the stock of the gun with his name and a date inscribed. James had written him a note that said: "Always remember this date. It was Labor Day, and as we waited in the field for the doves to come, you prayed and asked Jesus into your heart to be your Lord and Savior. That will always be the most important day of your life."

He continued "Mr. Wiggins led me to the Lord. Now my wife and children are Christians too. I have used and treasured that gun through the years. I have a wonderful family, and a good job now. The gun hangs over my fireplace in our den. I thank God every time I think about Mr. Wiggins." I thought, what a wonderful young man he was, and he was so kind to share with us.

Another friend (who lives near us) told how one Sunday morning, his wife had to go to Sunday School early, so James had given him a ride. He said that as they approached a traffic light, James gave him a dollar to give to the young man that was selling papers there. He asked James if we did not take the paper. James answered affirmatively, however he said that he had stopped one Sunday morning and talked with the young man. It seemed that his Dad had left the family. His mother was sick and had three younger children to care for. So he told James that he was selling papers on the week-ends to help his mother. Somehow, James knew of this family, through a mutual acquaintance. He told our friend that anytime a young man will get out in the heat and the cold as he had done for three years, he deserved an extra dollar each week. The friend embarrassed James by telling this at church. When James got home that day, he had shared this with me. He said, "I'm just glad that he didn't ride home with me and see me giving the crippled man on the returning corner a dollar."

Melany had helped Jake and me in planning James' funeral. One of the songs that she had chosen for Phillip Shepperd to sing was, "Thank You." The song describes a man dying and going to Heaven. There many souls came to him and thanked him for all the varied things that he had done for them. How appropriate for James.

Phillip also sang James' favorite hymn, "Victory in Jesus." Whether we sang it in church, heard it at home or in the car, when James heard the part that said, "How He made the lame to walk again, and caused the blind to see--" he would have tears in his eyes, and often running down his cheeks. He so wanted Melany to be able to walk again. But as difficult as it sometimes was, we always accepted God's sovereignty in all things.

Mark Harris (our former Pastor) from Charlotte and our assistant Pastor, Sherrell Dunn had James' service. It was beautiful.

Dear friends were pallbearers. Honorary pallbearers were James' IBEW Members, his Sunday School Class, and 10 Of Jake's friends. Many of the younger guys James had mentored and encouraged through the years. He prayed for all of them by name every day. It was not unusual for some of them to come by to see James, even when Jake was not there. He always loved young people, and they responded to him (and sometimes to his advice).

Mark reminded the young group (that he had known when he was here), that they had indeed lost a personal prayer warrior and a caring friend in James. He also said when he was our pastor that he always looked to the corner in the back of the sanctuary, where James always sat every service (I was not able to go to church with him for several years, because of caring for Melany). He said that he too had lost a prayer warrior and a partner.

Mark went on to tell how generous James was. How he never traded a car when we needed a newer one, but gave it to someone in need. With humor, he went on to tell a story a friend had related to him. He described how James called me to get a box and come out to my car, because we needed to clean it out. I knew that was odd, because James never cleaned out a car (everyone knew this and laughed). When I asked why are we doing this, James answered, "You know the little family (he called their name) in our neighborhood. The father has lost his job and cannot go for interviews because their car died. His wife is working a minimum wage job that barely feeds the family, and pays utilities. If he doesn't get work soon, they will lose their home."

I replied, "We don't have an extra car to give now." James said, "That's OK, Sweet, we'll get you another car when we can." Of course everyone laughed again, because they knew that was James.

One of the nicest things that Mark said about him was how deeply he loved and always took care of our family. How in difficult days he led us to chose Joy each day. That helped us all and others too.

It was a wonderful service. However, James would have been embarrassed by all the nice things that Mark said about him, and the heartfelt stories that we were told at the funeral home. He would have especially been uncomfortable with me writing all of this. He believed that when you did something in the name of the Lord, you should not tell anyone, just thank God that you could help and give Him the glory. On his bathroom mirror, he had pasted the scripture verse, Proverbs 19:19. The translation that he had copied said, *"He that giveth unto the poor, lendeth unto the Lord; and that which he hath given will God pay him again."* He often remarked, "Isn't it an humbling thing to think that we little finite beings can lend to the infinite Almighty God, who owns it all?"

He also had the verse, II Corinthians 9:7, *"Every man according as he purposeth in his heart, so let him give; not grudgingly, or of necessity; for God loveth a cheerful giver."* All of those that were near him, knew that he believed this, and humbly lived by it.

I have not shared these things about James to give the impression that he was a saint. He was far from that. But to let the people that shared things with us know how very much they have meant to my heart and to my family. And to thank them for reminding us that we too can be a blessing in small and large ways to others.

Melany was able to attend the service with her entourage of caretakers. That included a doctor, a nurse, her friend Stan, her two cousins, Darlene and Kimberly (who is also a nurse), as well as Tequila, our friend and wonderful helper. Toward the end of the service she stopped breathing and the alarm on her machine sounded. They all exited the side door with her. Jake left to help.

It was hard for me to remain in my seat. But I knew they could take care of her and handle the situation. I knew she would be upset if I followed. They got her breathing again and took her home. Jake came back for the remainder of the service.

The beautiful service concluded with the congregation singing, "Because He Lives." James was entombed in the Mausoleum next to Ric.

This was one of the poems on his funeral program. It appropriately described his philosophy and his faith.

SEE GOD IN ALL THINGS

See GOD in all things, great and small,
And give HIM praise whate're befall;
In life or death, in pain or woe,
See GOD and overcome thy foe.
I saw HIM in the morning light,
HE made the day shine clear and bright;
I saw HIM in the noontide hour,
And gained from HIM a refreshing shower.
At eventide, when worn and sad,
HE gave me help and made me glad.
At midnight, when on tossing bed,
My weary soul to sleep HE led.
I saw HIM when great losses came,
And found HE loved me just the same.
When heavy loads I had to bear,
I found HE lightened every care;
By sickness, sorrow, sore distress,
HE calmed my mind and gave me rest.
HE'S filled my heart with gladsome praise,
Since I gave HIM the upward gaze.

'Twas new to me, yet old to some,
The thought that to me has become;
A revelation of the way,
We all should live throughout the day;
For as each day unfolds its light,
We'll walk by faith and not by sight.
Life will indeed a blessing bring,

If we SEE GOD IN EVERYTHING!

A.E. Finn

Many beautiful sympathy cards were sent to us with touching messages. In the section of our newspaper they have a web site with a place to write condolences. Several wrote comforting notes. These all were indeed comforting and appreciated.

After her dad died Melany wrote these words for the plaque on the double marker in the Mausoleum where I will be entombed with James.

> *"When the Lord sent someone in need to them,*
> *They always sought to help and glorify Him."*

Many agreed that this summarized James' thoughts of life -- giving and taking care of others. I share most of his philosophy of giving to others, I just can't always afford it.

We all missed James so very much. We were truly thankful that he was indeed ready to die and that he was no longer suffering, physically, because of the cancer or emotionally because he could not take care of us.

We talked of how difficult his life had been for the last three months. Anyone that didn't see him could not have believed how hard it was for him. He had always been quite a talker, and so enjoyed talking to people. He had lost his voice seven months ago and could only whisper. As I had stated, he had lost one hundred and forty pounds, he only weighed one hundred pounds when he died.

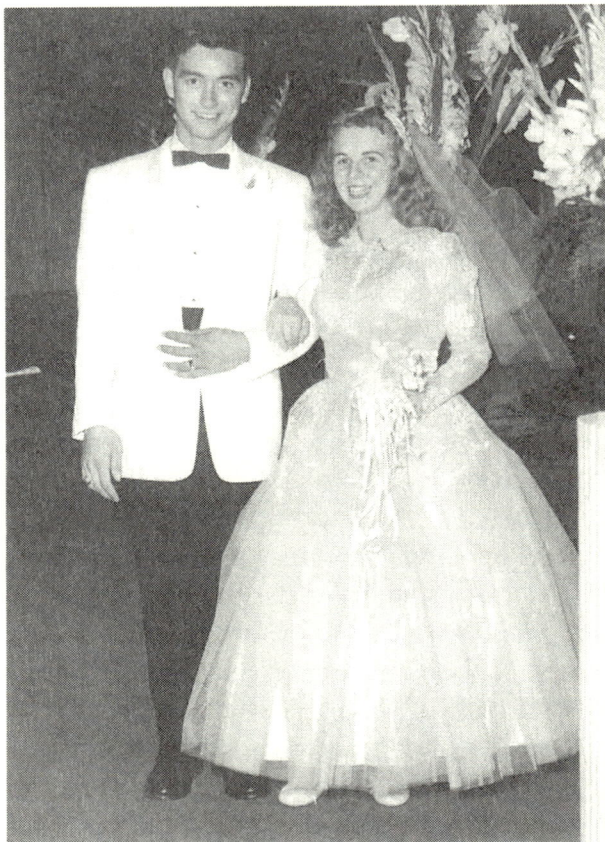

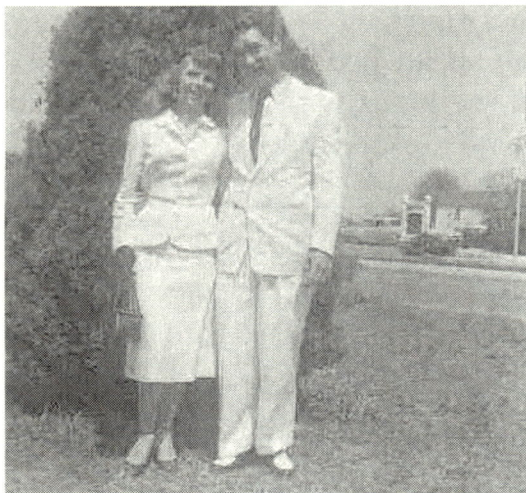

James and Nancy
on their wedding day
(top)
and in their white
"going-away suits"
in 1955 (left)

One of the saddest times we shared was concerning the week before Jake came home for the Christmas Holidays. It was during the time that I was sleeping one hour with James and one hour with Melany. About four a.m. I heard a consistent bumping noise through the living room wall. I thought it was the wind blowing the loose piece of siding. When I went out at five-thirty as I started over to check on James, I found that someone had trying to break into the sunroom door by removing the door facing. I didn't want to leave Melany in that situation so I waited until about six-thirty, after I gave Melany her morning medicine and daylight came before I left Melany. James was asleep when I got over there. He woke about seven thirty. I fixed his breakfast and waited for him to eat before I went back to Melany. She didn't usually wake back up until ten or eleven. I didn't tell either one of them about the attempted entry, I just called Don to come and fix it.

Around noon James wanted to go out on the patio that joins our condos and sit in the sun. Don had already repaired the door, and had just "dropped in" to see James. James noticed that the facing had been repaired because it was not painted. Of course he wanted to know what had happened. When I told him, he broke down and cried. He said, "Do you know how hard it is for me. After taking care of you and my family for fifty-three years. I am not strong enough to even begin to defend you anymore. This is the hardest part of my illness." He continued, "This, and not being able to witness for my Lord."

Tearfully, I assured him that the Lord had always sustained us and taken care of us in many difficult circumstances. I said, "You have always led me and the children to trust and rely on God. We will all continue to do this and we will be alright." It broke my heart to see him pained like that.

Jake recalled how hard it must have been when people didn't recognize him anymore. He also recanted how on the Saturday before he died on Sunday Night how he sat in his recliner and continually reached his hand for Jesus.

Melany recalled some real heart to heart talks that they had. She said he said many times how very proud he was of her and how he felt so badly that she had endured such a hard life. He told her that her life had touched many people and he was so glad that God had given her to us.

She said on their last talk, the Tuesday before his death they had shared, as they had many times before about Heaven and how wonderful it would be. He was so ready to go!

We knew we would always miss him, and our hearts would hurt forever until we were reunited with him. We agreed we were thankful that Jesus had reached down and took him to the wonderful place of peace and rest!

Beecher wrote:
"When the sun goes below the horizon he is not set, the heavens glow for a full hour after his departure.
And when a great and good man sets, the sky of this world is luminous long after he is out of sight.
Such a man cannot die out of the world. When he goes he leaves behind him much of himself, being dead, he speaks."

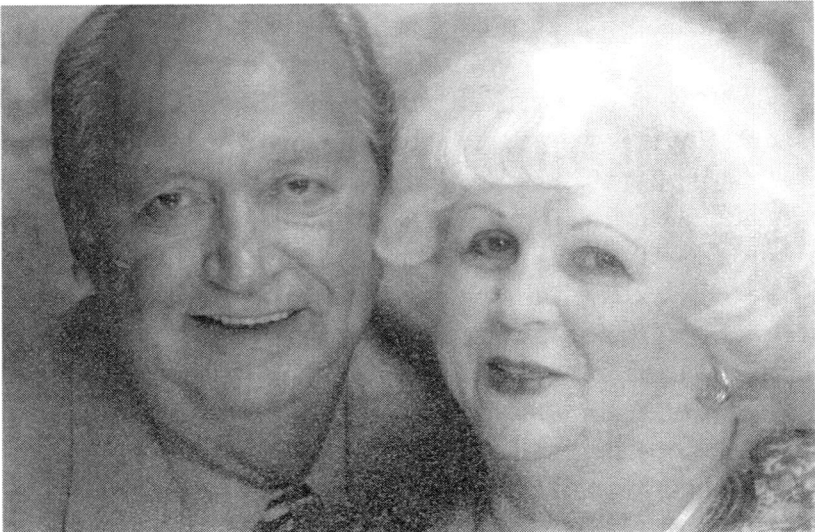

James and Nancy

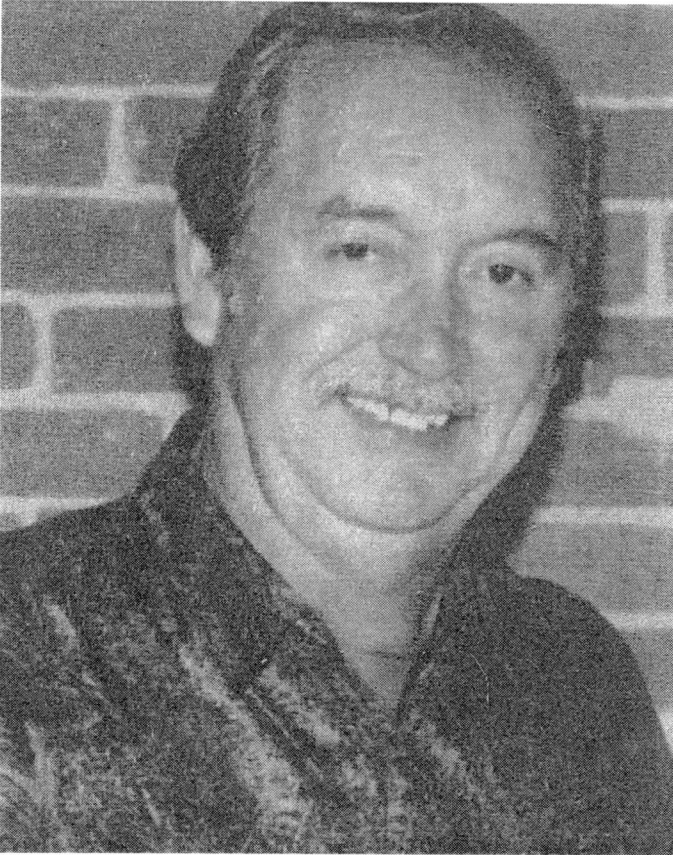

James

CHAPTER XV
PERFECT PEACE

"Thou wilt keep him in perfect peace,
Whose mind is stayed on thee;
Because he trusteth in thee."
Isaiah 26:3.

After James died, the rest of February was busy, but rather uneventful. Melany was very sad but didn't seem to be depressed. We continued the weekly trips to the hospital to get her Huber Needle changed and for them to give her the necessary IV Fluids, when she was able to go. When she couldn't make it to the hospital, the nurses came to her.

Friends came and stayed with Melany while Jake and I attended to the many hours of business associated with the days following a death. Melany and I were happy that Jake was home from college for that semester, he was a tremendous help to both of us.

Melany would go over to our condo when she was able, while Jake and I went through James' clothes and personal things. Of course Melany wanted to be there, because she always wanted to be in charge of everything. She was a lot of help, because organization was her strong forte. She laughingly said, that she wanted to be sure that she got the things of her Dad's that she wanted to keep. Most of his clothes, except the few things that Jake could wear, we took to the Homeless Mission that James was very involved with. The men there had their own stories to tell of how kind he was, how he always treated all of them with respect (many people don't) and he encouraged them in many ways.

Only ten days after James died was Valentine's Day. We celebrated very quietly. Several couple friends had invited me to go out with them, as we had many times in the past. My Valentine was gone and I just really wanted to be alone with my sweet memories. Melany's friend, Stan brought dinner and gifts for us. He was and is always so thoughtful, even to me today. Of course, Jake had his own plans.

February seventeenth was James' seventieth birthday. I had already rented a nice place in January, to have both of our families and many friends to come and celebrate with us.

Instead, Jake took me and Melany to her favorite seafood restaurant, to celebrate. Any eatery that had food was James' and Jake's favorite. We celebrated James' life and his birthday by sharing happy memories. We had so many. Melany was only able to eat a small amount, so we brought her meal home so she could enjoy it for several days. She often had to be suctioned when she ate, so she didn't want to subject the people eating near us to such a horrifying ordeal, if they were not used to it. It was hard, even if you were used to it. She never wanted to make anyone uncomfortable about anything.

I gave Jake the Tom-Tom (a GPS device) that I had bought for James. I realized then, how we had simply gone on planning for James to have a much longer life. In January James' cousins, Lucy and Ray had come up for a visit. They took James out to eat (some ordeal that was, I am sure), they could handle anything, and he enjoyed the outing very much. Ray had a Tom-Tom in his SUV. James wanted one just like it, because it was the first one that he had seen that he could see clearly and read easily. So, I went right out and bought him one for his birthday. He hadn't driven since Thanksgiving (two months). He could hardly walk without assistance. We had hope that he would be able to travel again. That was an unreasonable hope, but we could not turn loose of it.

In March Melany started planning for a trip to the beach in May, or maybe October. She said, "I'll hopefully be stronger by October." What an eternal hope and faith! The weather was mild, so we took Melany out to the lake and for several rides in the new van we had purchased after hers had died.

Friends continued visiting and Melany enjoyed this immensely. She had decided by the end of March that we probably should plan on going to St. Simons in October. She said that she knew she would feel better in the fall.

We started going through several boxes that we had stored for several years, most of it was Melany's "stuff" from High School and College. She enjoyed seeing things she had not seen for quite a while, and we had a lot of fun. We found some poems that she had written in 1984, when she was a Junior in High School. She was in the hospital for a very long time. Following, is one of them.

MY TRUE PURPOSE
I lay awake at night and wonder
what others are doing with their time,
It's a cinch it's probably not what I'm doing with mine.
They are running around, chasing dreams,
thinking their life's are sublime,
I'm laying here in bed, feeling terrible,
wondering if life for me-holds any reason or rhyme.
Is my life really worth anything--rolling around in a wheelchair and
being dependent on others?
Why must I be the one chosen to be different?-
I'd be like everyone else, if I had my
"I'd rathers,"
So, why exactly did God choose for me to be His "different" one?
Why did He choose for me to sit, rather than to walk or run?
I believe my God holds the answer,
and I believe He'll reveal it to me,
It may not be in this lifetime, but someday
He'll make it clear why it must be.
I mustn't be too anxious--that's a lesson to be heeded,

I'm really working on patience--I know this
time of rest is needed.
I can be a beacon for Christ, and share with
others His wonderful name.
Or, I can be bitter and resentful and on that
same name bring shame.
The former is better and much more so, the
latter would be a sin,
For my true purpose, like everyone else's, is
to share Him with my fellow men."

Melany Wiggins
April 21, 1984

She asked, "Do you really think that my life has helped anyone?" I assured her that it had. Then I sighted several examples people had expressed to me.

We also read the account of her dream of Heaven when her heart had stopped twice in 2004, while she was hospitalized. Melany said, "If your heart stops, it is good to be in the hospital so they can help immediately." My thoughts exactly. She continued "It was wonderful to dream about how beautiful Heaven will be. I can't wait to get there and see my Jesus, my Daddy, Ric, Greg, and my baby sisters. Won't it be wonderful?"

* * * * *

This is her dream just as she told it to me at 3 a.m. and 6 a.m., each time she started breathing again. I wrote it in my notebook and typed it later. Both accounts were identical.

MELANY WIGGINS
Tuesday, February 2, 1999
3 a.m. and 6 a.m.

"I came to a beautiful crystal clear river (with a slight blue tinge). There was the most beautiful bridge going over the river. The bridge had many vibrant colors and was outlined in bright gold.

There were animals made of gold sitting on the sides of the bridge. The road on the bridge was soft pastel colors streaked with gold. It was SO pretty. I floated (or slowly flew) over the bridge. As I passed over, the animals came to life. There were hummingbirds, many butterflies, several different birds, and miniature cats, dogs, and even horses. They fluttered and flew in front of me and all around me. It felt as though I was surrounded by love.

As I floated over the bridge, I came to a tunnel made out of gold. As I started into the tunnel I looked back, because the animals had left me. They were back on the bridge in statue form in their brilliant gold.

The tunnel was so inviting. It was filled with the most marvelous pastel colors I have ever seen. The colors swirled and floated in streaks like a kaleidoscope turning. As I entered the tunnel, the colors brushed me like soft clouds. It felt so peaceful. As I slowly floated through, the tunnel slowly narrowed, the feeling was wonderful and serene. I was drawn back out of the tunnel and I woke up. I never made it through."

Melany could repeat this account verbatim for the doctors and nurses, as they came to hear it. Later, she added--"I know this must be a glimpse of what Heaven is like....Beautiful, but it will be so much more grand when I see my Lord Jesus and my many loved ones."

The last week of April 2008, actually according to the notes in my spiral notebook, it was April 13, one month before she died on May 13th. Melany had two dreams, on consecutive nights. Each was similar, she dreamed that she was dying. She and I went over her salvation experience that had occurred when she was seven years old. She said that she knew that it was real, she just wanted to be sure. Once again she stated, "When Jesus is ready for me, I'm ready for Him."

She wanted to watch the CD of her Dad's funeral service. She told me then that she wanted her funeral service to be just like his. She asked me to choose the poems that I felt would be appropriate to have in her order of service. I had already thought of several through the years that described her life. I found them in my devotional book, and shared them with her. She said, "People always say such nice things about me. I just want my funeral service to honor Christ and point others to Him!

Melany didn't seem to be depressed, she just was reflective. But I'm sure that she knew that my health was not the best at that time. James and I had always planned how she would be cared for, if something happened to me. James had never been sick, and even the doctors were surprised that he died first.

The first week in May, Melany said, "Mother, I want you to do something for me. Please pray that I will die before you do. No one else could ever take as good of care of me, as you have."

I answered with tears in my heart and eyes, "Melany, I cannot pray for you, my child, to die. But, I will pray that God will honor and answer your prayers, whatever they may be. If it is in accordance with His will"

I asked Jake to come over and I shared the plans and arrangements that James and I had made for her, and for Jake to always be taken care of. Through careful planning there was enough money to take care of them, since her medicines of over twenty-thousand dollars per month were now covered under Medicaid.

Melany reminded me, that when her Dad died, she and I both had received an increase in our monthly checks. She was afraid that now they would take her Medicaid away. I already knew that this was a real possibility, but I had not voiced it to anyone.

I assured her that the Lord had always taken care of us, reminding her of the other financial difficulties we had in the past. That He had then provided more, in financial blessings.

She had her own condo, with a guest room for a full-time caretaker to live in. There was plenty to pay for all her needs. Four friends had assured us that they would always see that her needs were met, and that she could stay in her own place. She had five cousins (and their precious spouses) here in Augusta that would all help look after her. Plus other family members offered their help and support for her after I was gone.

Jake assured her that he would always stay in my other two condos (connected with a door, making it an eight room house), right next door. He was as capable of taking care of Melany as I was. She trusted him explicitly.

During the following days, we reread the manuscript for her book and shared some of it with several friends and family members. She told me one week before she died that she wanted me to promise her that I would type her book, and get it published. She said, I just want it to glorify Jesus. I had hand written it in a large spiral notebook. She had dictated some of it, as we shared ideas, thoughts and memories at the beach in 2006.

Of course, we had not planned to write the manuscript while we were at the beach, so we had some difficulty recalling certain things and dates. She was much better at this than I was. When we returned home, I got out my collection of "spiral notebooks," that I use as a "sometime" journal. My family and friends had often laughed at me because anything they wanted to know, I had in my notebooks. I just couldn't find it sometimes. I assured her that I would try to finish it and have it published.

Melany was getting much weaker. There were difficult days when she struggled to breathe, even on the breathing machine. She was just so tired. When friends called to come for a visit, she said that she just didn't feel like having company to-day, please call back in a few days.

After Melany's death, one of my friends visited me. She read one of the many little plaques that were in Melany's condo. It said "Laughter is the music of the heart." She commented, "Melany loved her Dad so much. When he died, it was if the music left her heart."

Then I realized some things that I had not thought of. Melany loved music all of her life. It was as though music was her life at times. She played her CD's and tapes all the time. She had a five CD changer in the cabinet by her bed, with many discs next to it.

She had been given the gracious privilege of meeting "backstage" after two of their concerts in Augusta, two of her favorite singers. They were Amy Grant and Sandi Patti, I believe she had all of their CD's, and had played them daily. She had also met Joni Erickson Tada when we attended a seminar she and her husband Ken, conducted in Columbia, S.C.

We had a room next to them in the motel. She was able to spend some quality time with them, a real joy to her. She had Joni's CD's as well.

It occurred to me that she had hardly played any music since her Dad died. It really seemed as though the music really had gone out of her life and heart. How could I have not noticed this?

* * * * *

Tuesday, May 13th, 2008, was one of the longest (although it ended all too quickly), hardest days of my entire life. It started on Monday night the 12th. I always taped our Sunday morning worship service at Curtis Baptist. Jake had not gone to services on Sunday morning, so I invited him and his college friend, Jason, to come over Monday night and watch the service with Melany and me. Melany never watched anything until early afternoon, then well into the night.

They came over and watched as two of Jake's friends sang a duet. Then our wonderful music director, Phillip Shepperd sang, "I Can Only Imagine." The song so beautifully describes Heaven and what awaits us there. When he finished the song, Melany said, "I just wish Jesus would come and get me now, I am so ready to go to Heaven."

Jason looked at her with a startled expression on his face, I don't believe he had ever heard anyone say that they wanted to go to Heaven to-day.

The service continued with a guest minister, Dr. Pike from Atlanta, Ga. He presented a great sermon, directed at young people. Jason had not been raised in the church, so when the message closed, he began asking questions about some things that he had heard. Jake and I answered a few.

Melany asked Jason to pull his chair close to her bed, then she began to share with him, what God meant to her and how He had sustained her through the many years of sickness and suffering. She was so very short of breath, she would have to pull her mask down so that he could hear her. Jason listened very patiently and attentively. She said, "Jason, don't you want to know Jesus personally and have Him in your heart and Life?" Jason answered affirmatively. Then she led him in the sinner's prayer, that he repeated after her. When they finished, she said, "Jason, you have accepted Jesus as your Lord and Savior, now you will join me and Papa (he loved James very much), in Heaven." By then, she was completely exhausted, breathing heavily, and drenched in perspiration. The guys went back over to Jake's.

After they left, I got her something to drink, wiped her face, neck and arms with a cool cloth. She said, "Mother, this is the last witness I will ever be able to give for my wonderful Lord." I replied, "I surely hope not." She said, "That's Okay. Do you remember that I asked you a few days ago, if you thought that when we have completed the tasks that God had placed us here for, He would take us home to Heaven? This may be my last thing that God has planned for me to do."

I did remember, I had answered at that time that I was not sure if those words were Biblical or not, but the Scripture says that there is an appointed time unto man to die. We had many conversations about death, dying and Heaven during the last month. I had felt, it was because of her Dad's death, that so much was on her mind. I thought of these conservations all during that last night.

Melany was very tired, but she didn't go to sleep, because she was gasping for breath. She had asked me to replay Phillip's song, "I Can Only Imagine," several times. I thought that she had stopped breathing, about three o'clock Tuesday morning. I called Jake, and of course he came immediately. He was strong enough to do as James had done many times for her to help her breathe. He would stand beside her, put his hands on her back, under her lungs and lift up and down. Since her diaphragm didn't work properly, it would help her to breathe. After he got her breathing again, Jake laid down behind her back (we had her hospital bed as straight up as it would go), so that his body pushed against her back. The many pillows did not support her lungs, like his body did. He stayed in that strained position for the rest of the night.

Melany and I never went to sleep. By daylight, she was breathing easier. I told Jake to go to his house and get some sleep, I would call him if necessary.

She normally took her Medication, Oxycotin at 7 a.m. and 7 p.m. I took her small pill to her, and she said that she didn't need it, that she wasn't in pain just now, and had rather wait until later.

She was hardly talking at all, which was very unusual for her. Although, as I have mentioned, she didn't do mornings well. I knew she was very tired. About nine o'clock I asked her if I could call Dr. Jones and ask him if she could come to the hospital and get some fluid, maybe it would make her feel better. She answered, "Mother it will probably make you feel better." Then she asked me very matter of factually, "Mother, why are you fighting this?" I couldn't answer. However, she said that she would go if he wanted her to, but she would not stay.

I called our dear Dr. Jones, who had tried so hard through the years to make her life easier, as had all of the doctors. He had arranged on Friday for Hospice to start coming on Tuesday. They had already called me for a pre-phone interview.

Dr. Jones said that he would be glad for her to come and see if he could do anything, but that fluid was building around her heart, and adding more fluids could possibly cause more problems. He suggested that I call Dr. Joseph, our Pulmonary Doctor.

Dr Joseph said that IF she would agree to a ventilator, and we both knew she would not, it would be hard to intubate her because she was completely "sandwiched" over. Both doctors checked with us throughout the day.

Unexpectedly, one of her doctors came to the house, during his lunchtime. He is a fine Christian. I stayed in the Living Room and let him check her. They talked for a while, then he prayed with her. When he came into the living room, he asked Jake and me step out into the sunroom. There he told us, something we probably knew but couldn't accept. He said that she will probably die within twelve hours. Then he kindly asked, "Are you two going to be alright? Can I call someone to come?" We assured him that we would be fine.

Jake asked, "Are you sure, you know they have told us several times to call the family in." With tears in his eyes, the doctor said that he was sure. He said she was completely in God's hands now, and she was ready to go, but not to the hospital.

After he left, we went back into Melany's room. She seemed totally at peace, our hearts were in turmoil. I told her that during the last week several friends had called and asked to see her. I asked her if she wanted me to call anyone. She said, no. I reminded her that Pastor Dunn had asked us to call him when she was able to have company. She said, "You can call them all tomorrow." I don't know if she knew that she would not be here tomorrow. She did not sleep, but she was still and quiet with her eyes closed most of the time. Jake and I would stay with her at all times.

One time, as I went into the kitchen to get her a cool drink (which she refused), I motioned for Jake to follow me. When I was sure that we were far enough away that Melany could not hear, I asked Jake, "Son, do you realize that we are just waiting for the Death Angel to come?" He nodded, then he asked, "How do you think we will do?" I couldn't speak. I responded by just slowly shaking my head. It was simply too much to grasp. But I knew that God was so close in all of our hearts, and he would see us through.

During the entire day, we had watched and felt as Melany's body grew colder. It started in her fingers and slowly traveled up her arms. By six o'clock it had reached her neck.

Brenda, Melany's hospital nurse who was also our dear friend from church, stopped by after work. She offered to stay with us, but I told her we would be alright. I just wanted to be with Melany and hold her frail little body as the warmth was leaving it.

That day Melany had not had any additional medicine except the Buprenex, the medicine that flowed continually from her cad pump, into her heart. She had refused all food except a few bites of frozen yogurt. She thought that she could drink a blue misty earlier, but when Jake went and got it, she drank very little.

* * * * *

On Monday night, after Jake and Jason had left, I had read to Melany from "Streams In the Desert." This was our favorite devotional book. The scripture verse for this date was, Mark 9:23. It said, *"All things are possible to him that believeth."* Melany struggled to breath, as she said, "This verse is really true. I have prayed for Jason since he became Jake's friend at college. I have claimed this verse for his salvation, and tonight we saw him saved. God is so good."

Early on Tuesday morning, and a couple of times throughout the day, she had asked me to reread that verse, and the devotion for that day. The verse of scripture for that date was Romans 8:26. It said, *"We know not what we should pray for as we ought."* It was so true for my heart, I didn't want my child to suffer anymore, but I didn't want to give her up, even to Jesus, not yet. But I did want the Lord's will to be done. The last of the devotional reading said:

"The way to peace and victory is to accept every circumstance, every trial, straight from the hand of a loving Father, and to live up in the heavenly places, above the clouds, in the very presence of the throne, and to look down from the glory upon our environment as lovingly and divinely appointed." -Selected- **STREAMS IN THE DESERT**

Melany and I always watched the sunset out of the window by her bed. She would start watching about eight o'clock. This time of the year it usually set about eight-thirty. We kept her blind up so she could see all of its beauty over the lake that she loved so much.

Jake was outside by her window watering her flowers. She had me call him to come in. She told him, "One of the nicest things that I have enjoyed the most, besides having my own condo, is the beautiful flower garden that you planted and tend for me. I appreciate it very much, with the fountain and the bird feeders to enjoy constantly."

Jake smiled and nodded, then went out to finish his watering. Melany asked me to sing all the stanzas of Jesus Loves Me. I did, but I don't know how I did it. She asked me to repeat the last stanza, *"Jesus loves me, He will stay, close beside me all the way. If I love Him when I die, He will take me home on high."*

She simply smiled, then asked me to read the passage from the Bible that we always read before she faced the many surgeries. I had read it to her a couple of times during the night. Psalm 121 tells of God's sustaining power. It begins in verse one, *"I will lift up mine eyes unto the hills, from whence cometh my help."* It continues by saying, *"God never slumbers nor sleeps, He always watches over us."* The last verse says, *"The Lord shall preserve thy going out and thy coming in from this time forth, and even for evermore."*

She then asked me to sing all the verses of "Amazing Grace."

Somehow I stumbled through that. I was holding her hands, she could no longer move them. But just as her Dad had tried to do, she responded to the last stanza, by moving her index finger as I sobbing sang, *"When we've been there ten thousand years, bright shining as the sun. We've no less days to sing God's praise than when we first begun."* I hugged her and cried, "Baby, I love you so much, I don't want you to go." She smiled and weakly said, "I know, but I must."

Just as the sun set, she regained amazing strength, and said, "Look God gave me a beautiful 'Cotton-Candy' sunset." That was always her favorite kind of sunset, where the glow of the sun left colors of pink, purple, blue and some yellow. Then she said, "Just think how beautiful it is from Heaven." Earlier, I had pulled my wheelchair close to the bed. I had placed my left arm around her frail little body (now she only weighed 60 pounds). I had my right hand covering hers, suddenly, she said "Oh! Oh!" I asked, "Am I hurting you?" "No! No!" she strongly replied, "Jesus! Jesus! I see Jesus!" Then she was gone!

My heart was broken. But any mother would rejoice that her child went straight from her loving arms into the precious, everlasting arms of Jesus.

* * * * *

After Melany died, I sat in total shock for several minutes. The bells and whistles were sounding loudly, and I still just sat there, waiting for her to start back breathing. Finally, while I still had her cradled in my arms, I felt of her neck, that was already cold. I did not cry, I just waited. As I looked out of the window, I saw Jake put the hose down and go around the back of the condo. Thinking that he was coming in the sunroom door, I went into the living room to meet him. Bradley, Don, Nate and Jason (all Jake's friends) were coming in the back door ahead of Jake, who had probably stopped to turn off the hose. Jake had not heard the machines going off from outside. Bradley said, "Nana, Jake told us how very sick Mimi is, and we just wanted to come by and tell her that we are thinking about her and we love her." He had brought her a blue misty drink.

Then, I started to cry and asked the guys to let Jake come on in ahead of them. As I was telling Jake that I thought Melany was gone, he heard the blaring noise and ran past us into her bedroom. We could hear him calling to her as he silenced the machines warnings.

I went into the room to remind him that Melany had made us promise several times that if she died at home that we would not turn off the machines immediately, and would not call the funeral home for at least two hours. She wanted to be sure that she was really dead. James had made the same request. Jake hugged me, and said, "Nana, she is really gone."

The friends were sitting in the living room, I still remember that picture vividly, some were crying, the others were trying not to. I stood in the doorway and told them that they could come into her room and see her, if they wanted to. But if they didn't feel comfortable doing this, it was alright. They all came into the room, looked at her, and some told her that they loved her, some uttered something quietly. Then they went back into the living room and sat down, some were crying. I don't think any of them had witnessed death before. They were all very reflective. Then they left.

Bradley had called his mom, she had called her friend (Alisha), Roy's secretary for her to call Joyce and Roy. Joyce called immediately, and asked if they could come. I told her not yet, I would let her know, but she could call Pat and Buddy.

I still did not believe that Melany was really gone. It was as though, if I let people start coming then I would be acknowledging that she was really dead. She had stopped breathing several times before and would start back in a few seconds or minutes. Jake and I just sat in stunned silence. Then I started crying uncontrollably. I continued hugging her, and begging the Lord, to not take her now.

Jake had a little more presence of mind and thoughts. He started calling people. We called Dr. Jones, he said we could call the funeral home and they would send the coroner (since she had died at home), before they came to get her body.

My mind is very cloudy concerning the next few hours. Our friends all started coming. I moved back and forth from the living room to the bedroom, still checking to see if she had started back breathing. Finally, they told me I had to call the funeral home (a couple hours had passed). Time seemed to stand still for me.

The coroner came, and we turned off the machines. I knew that our coroner was out of town, and this was an assistant. I found out later, that he was a retired military man, and this was one of his first home visits. He was very business-like, and almost rude. As I moved to the bed to take the Huber needle out of Melany's chest, he stopped me. Jake had turned off the cad pump, but the Heparin drip mixed in the bag of fluid was "piggy-backed" into one port, with the Buprenex going into another. The coroner grabbed the scissors off of the bedside table and cut the line from the Heparin and fluids that were connected. Immediately the fluids gushed out, all over Melany and me. Then he told me, rather curtly to move back. He examined her body, and asked some questions about her health, and what had happened at her time of death. Then he asked why we had waited so long to call him.

Jake explained Melany's wishes for us to wait a couple of hours. She had died at eight-thirty, and it was ten-thirty now. He did not seem at all happy with the answer.

The gentleman asked about her medicine. Jake got it for him. We kept it in a basket on the entertainment center, across the room. He asked if she had access to her medicines. We told him, that I gave her the medicines. When I was not available, then Jake gave them to her. Very seldom did anyone else give them. He asked for the names of the others that had access to her medicines, as the basket contained strong medications. We explained that she did not take all of the medicines every day. He wanted to know from me, the last time any had been given, and what they were. I felt like I was really being interrogated.

Although I realized later that these were probably standard procedures, it was surprising and a little frightening to me at that time, as though he thought I had done something wrong. Jake asked him why did he need to know all of this at this time, because I was becoming upset. Our friends were all sitting in the living room listening to all of this in silence. As the man said, "We just always have to be sure that there is no foul play." Roy, who is very calm in most circumstances, rose from his chair. He informed him that this was a well-loved, and well-cared for young lady for many years, and that nothing wrong had been done here. The coroner said OK.

By then the funeral director had arrived. The coroner said that they had to wait for the EMT's to come and pronounce her dead. We thought that was what the coroner did. Soon the ambulance arrived with the EMT's, followed by the fire truck, the rescue truck and the police. The house was full, and it was all very confusing, as we had to give information to all of them, except the firemen.

Finally, they all left except the funeral home director, and our many friends. I watched in horror from the living room doorway, as they bagged her precious little body. With her body completely drawn over, and her legs missing, I had an uncanny thought that she looked about the size of a large dog. Jake moved me from the doorway, so they could pass. As I sobbed, I begged them not to take her yet! Joyce and Roy walked out with Jake and they watched them load her body into the hearse.

I don't remember much else that happened. I am recanting this part of her death and the following hours for one reason only. Hopefully it will be a comfort to those that go through similar situations, to not judge themselves or their actions to harshly, as they react to the death of a loved one.

Many of our friends have seen me go through some very difficult situations for many years. They have always commented how they felt I could handle any situation, they found out differently that night, as I completely fell apart. There is no right or wrong way to handle yourself at the time of the death of a loved one. There is no protocol or etiquette; for each situation is different, and each person handles themselves differently.

My grief was overwhelming. I had just started this painful journey with James' death. My heart had not even begun to start the healing process dealing with the grief of losing my husband just three months ago.

Friends started leaving around midnight. Several offered to stay with me, others made us promise that we would call them if we needed anything.

Jake and I talked briefly, then I told him to go on over to his condo and get some rest. I would be alright, and I needed some time alone. Reluctantly, he left.

I took the sheets off of Melany's hospital bed, and placed a quilt over the air mattress that was still inflated and was rotating the air. I climbed up on the bed. She slept with a soft brown dog that Ric had given her on his last visit with her. Dr. Dennis had given her a bear (she named it Dr. D) on her birthday, during one of her lengthy hospital stays. I took the two stuffed animals and cuddled them to my chest. It was comforting, they still smelled like her. As exhausted as I was, I still could not go to sleep. I just couldn't turn my mind and thoughts off.

I was so tired, and I felt that I was really just dreaming, and I would surely wake up at any moment. Then reality set in, I cried until I had no tears. I asked the Lord to just please take me now, tonight.

I knew from things I had learned in teaching and experiencing grief that the worst was yet to come. It seems that the Lord gives us a feeling of numbness for the first few days, and sometimes for weeks. We could not stand all of the grief at once. I wasn't sure that I could go through this again. I picked up Melany's Bible from the bedside table and began to read some verses that she had marked. God's word is always a comfort in time of any need, especially sorrow. I relived the last few weeks and days in my mind and heart.

I do not know if Melany saw the Death Angel or not, but I'm sure she saw Jesus. I thought of the time in the hospital four years ago when she asked me to call Mark and ask him to please pray, and ask Jesus to come to her hospital window on the white cloud, riding the white horse he was talking about, and get her. I'm sure she saw it all. I got up and found the song that she had often heard our church sing on the TV.

She had written the words in her spiral notebook.

"Behold He comes, riding on a cloud,
Shining like the sun, at the trumpets call;
Lift your voice, it's the year of Jubilee and
Out of Zion's hills salvation comes."

I'm sure she was happy with all the wonders that she enjoyed, with her Dad and Ric and Greg, her little sisters and her beloved grandparents.

I thanked God truly, from my heart for taking her and James out of their pain and sickness. I told Him I knew that He could and would help me get through these next few busy days of preparation for the funeral; to please give me clarity of mind. Also, to let Melany's funeral glorify Him. My trust was in Him, for I knew I could not do it on my own. Then I had a few hours of restful sleep.

*   *   *   *

I got off of the bed (it was quite high), made my coffee, and read my devotion for the day. It closed with a pointed poem by Annie Johnson Flint, directed straight to my heart:

"I prayed for strength, and then I lost awhile
All sense of nearness, human and divine;
The love I leaned on failed and pierced my heart.
The hands I clung to loosed themselves from mine;
But while I swayed, weak, trembling, and alone,
The everlasting arms upheld my own.
I prayed for light; the sun went down in clouds,
The moon was darkened by a misty doubt.

The stars of Heaven were dimmed by
earthly fears.
And all my little candle flames burned out;
But while I sat in shadow, wrapped in night,
The face of Christ made all
The darkness bright.
I heard His voice and had
Perfect Peace.
Giver of good, so answer each request,
With thine own giving, better than my best."

I knew now, that I could make it through these days, weeks, months and years. I just had to take them day by day, sometimes hour by hour, and maybe minute by minute, always step by step, trusting God to lead me. I knew I would stumble, face fears I had never know, falter and at times fail. But with Jesus in my heart and life, I could make it.

I felt refreshed and renewed, a feeling that vacillated between that feeling and the feeling of tiredness and exhaustion many times in the days, weeks and months ahead.

I remembered a little verse I had often quoted:
"The heart that loves and serves and sings,
Hears everywhere the _whisper_ of angels wings."
(STREAMS IN THE DESERT says _rush_)

Indeed, I had been blessed for many years and in many situations by feeling the 'whisper' of angels' wings in my heart."

Roger and Rosa arrived early that morning. We began the familiar journey, made some calls, called Mark Harris to see when he could come for the service. Then we went to the funeral home to make the final arrangements. Some things were a little easier this time.

Melany had stated that she wanted a white casket with pink lining. She wanted the praying hands corners that were on her

Dad's, replaced with Angels. She wanted to be buried in the white dress that she had worn in her Coronation Ceremony when she was crowned "Queen Regent In Service,, as a teenager. She had even had me try it on her several weeks ago. Then she had said, "I want to wear this beautiful dress again, when I really have my Coronation Ceremony in Heaven."

In retrospect, we realized that Melany apparently knew she was going to her Heavenly Home soon. She was preparing for her long awaited journey. She was trying to prepare us as well. How could I have missed this? So many things I have wished I had done for her. So many things I have wished I had said to her. If I had only been more aware. The arrangements went beautifully, according to her wishes.

Once again, we filled the Hotel near our home as family and friends began arriving. Our church family and friends filled our home with food and our hearts with kindness and love.

We had the visitation at the funeral home for two nights. Once again many came with encouragement, sharing thoughts and stories about Melany. Many were quite humorous, some very tender and others shared that Melany had made a profound impact on their lives, some even life-changing!

How dear all of these things were to our hearts. In the weeks ahead the visits, cards, messages and comments in our newspaper memorials were heart rending, but very encouraging and much appreciated.

The day of Melany's funeral, our church family fed our large family lunch, before the service. Her funeral was indeed Christ Honoring, just as she had requested. The touching music was beautifully sung by Phillip Shepherd, including "Victory in Jesus," "Beulah Land," and "Thank You." Then the congregation sang "Because He Lives." Our long-time friend, Joanne Farr (one of Melany's "Other Mothers"), the mother of her good friend Kimberly, sang "Amazing Grace," at the Committal Service at the Mausoleum. She had also done this when James and Ric were entombed.

Dr. John Bryan was our pastor most of Melany's life. He

gave a beautiful message of their spiritual walk together. He was the pastor that was with her through all of her GA and Acteen Steps, and through her school years. He told of how difficult her life had been because of her disease, and he shared precious times that they had shared.

Melany had enjoyed John's family and shared many times with him, his dear wife Clare, and their three fine boys.

Dr. Mark Harris became our pastor after Melany had graduated from College. Melany loved him and his sweet wife Beth, and their family. They had two sons and one daughter. Jake was in their daughter Laura's class at school. John, the oldest son had played sports with Jake. The youngest, Matthew was active in sports also, so she enjoyed times with all of them.

Mark presented a wonderful, heartfelt message. He too told of several incidents that he and Melany had shared. He had known her well, during the latter part of her illness. He told of how she endured with great unwavering faith. Both pastors did an excellent job of their observing her as she expressed her faith and trust in the Lord. Also, both told of her care and interest in others and their problems.

The order of service sheet had printed the poem that she had written entitled, "My True Purpose." Also, a poem I had saved that described her life so well. It is at the end of this chapter. I'm sorry that the author is unknown, for it was truly written from their heart.

After the service many family members and friends came to the house. The local newspaper had written several articles about Melany. They had sent a reporter to her memorial service. That evening, they called and interviewed me. The next day they ran a very inspiring column about her.

Rev. Sherrell Dunn conducted the Committal Service at the Mausoleum. He and Melany had a very special relationship. He did a wonderful service.

She was entombed with her brother.

Ric's bronze marker reads:

"To well loved to ever be forgotten."

Melany's says:

"JOY she gave,
    PEACE she found.
Now she has JOY and PEACE forever
With Christ Jesus."

"How do we count the lives she touched,
    the light she shed for years?
How do we see the difference she made,
    when we're looking through our tears?

How do we know the things that are,
    that never should have been,
Without her valiant heart,
    that dared to fight and fight again?

How do we know what flowers will bloom
    from seeds of yesterday,
What songs are sung and dreams begun
    because she passed this way?

How do we measure the shining places
    that time can never pale,
In all the hearts that cheered her on
    and willed her to prevail?

How did her spirit soar beyond
    the suffering and the scars,
To live with one hand clutching hope
    and the other on the stars?

We may not know what she left behind
    on the difficult path she trod,
But we know this much:

Her life's brief touch,
was from the hand of God."

AUTHOR UNKNOWN

After Melany died, I found this poem in her Bible--it was dated August 6, 1992--She was in college at that time--I believe at this time she was at home for several months after a lengthy hospitalization.

DARKNESS

Darkness, choking, all consuming, Life averting.
What lives in the darkness? Fear, anger, and death. Smothering. Ever attempting to steal the new joy of dawn,
The fresh dew of morning, the bright glare at noontime.
Evening, growing ever darker, looming, longing to devour.
It waits for no one.
It seeks, it seeks, always hiding over the horizon. Suppressed.
But only briefly, for night must always come.
Yet, when the sky is darkest, the stars shine.
Ever brighter, casting shadows, not of fear, but of strength and might.
FOR WHEN THE SON SHINES,
the stars remain but cannot be seen.
Drawing strength from the SONLIGHT during the day;
they beam to their fullest in the midst of night.
In some small way giving the Son's light to the darkness,
in a burst of fire, glory, beauty and hope.
HOPE FOR A NEW DAY!
For no night endures forever.
No matter how bleak, desolate and difficult the night-morning will come.
Morning always comes. Fresh and new. Full of hope.
For everything is possible at daybreak.
IF YOU SURVIVE THE NIGHT!

(I'm just a star of the night. I pray that I gleamed, even for a little while, just for a moment!)
[All who knew her will attest that she did!]

Later I found this FROM EVENING THOUGHTS--It would surely have been an answer to her prayer that she did indeed glow for a little while--

"When we are called aside and can only suffer; when we are sick; when we are consumed wit6h pain; when all our activities have been dropped, we feel we are no longer of use, that we are not doing anything.

But, if we are patient and submissive, it is almost certain that we are a greater blessing to the world in our time of suffering and pain than we were in the days when we thought we were doing the most of our work. We are burning now, and shining because we are burning.

"Many want the glory without the cross, the shining without the burning, but crucifixion comes before coronation."

What a wonderful, glorious coronation awaited Melany in Glory!!

CHAPTER XVI
PERSONAL PEACE

"Come unto me, all ye that labor and are heavy laden, and I will give you rest." Matthew 11:28

I wanted this book to be only about God, others, Melany and James. However, as I have shared my testimony of God's grace to our family in our many times of need and distress many have asked me to write a book. When I finished this manuscript, I was asked to write a "brief" chapter on how I had personally handled these many situations in our lives for so many years.

Those who know me, know that I don't know how to do "brief" anything. To be brief, I could simply answer this question briefly. Some days good, some days bad! Now, how did I seek (always with God's help and the help of others) to turn the bad days into good? Sometimes yes, sometimes no!

However, there is a little more to it than that. I have many times pondered this question that has been asked. Without seeming redundant here, as I have said in many previous chapters, we all always acknowledged God as our main source of help and comfort. I would be amiss, if I did not also add the real contributions that others provided to us that helped me and our family through the often difficult days, months and years. The many doctors, and other medical professionals, our dear friends, our precious family and the many unknown (to us) people who prayed for us, all provided encouragement and strength so desperately needed. These people will never know this side of Heaven how often our faith was faltering and weak when we would receive a card, a call or visit that enabled us to go on trusting our Heavenly Father.

Now I have a real answer. After much prayer, meditation and contemplation, it is a very simple answer, with a very complex meaning of faith, it is simply we always believed in "The Sovereignty of God." I always share this, whether speaking in churches or sharing with individuals. James and I read, well I read and shared with him (that's how he liked to read), a book by Peg Rankin and her husband concerning how to handle difficult situations in life. They had taught an extensive class, lasting almost a year, dealing with the complexity of the Sovereignty of Almighty God. At the end of the class, they asked the members to write what they had learned and believed the Sovereignty of God really was. One young man, who acknowledged not being the "brightest" student wrote the following:

The Sovereignty of God:

God made us,
He always cares for us.
He has a purpose for our lives.
Therefore--
God has the right to do:
Anything He wishes to do,
Anytime He wants to do it,
Anyway He desires to do it,
For any purpose He seeks to accomplish.

I sincerely believe this with all my heart. I have seen it accomplish many things that I would have thought impossible. As I told in one of the previous chapters, we had decided without question that Melany's illness was to be used to glorify God. With the many acknowledgements of lives changed, expressions of encouragement, and of faith strengthened through her life, we know it was true.

Though I have not always understood what God was doing, I believed the young man's theory. However, when we went through the times of our son, Ric's addiction to drugs, and the consequences that followed, it was hard to believe that anything good could ever come out of it. It was one of the hardest times of our lives, because it was hard to see God in it.

One evening we were watching the mud-slides on television seeing trees, cars and houses, often with a chimney sticking up or part of a roof floating by. James commented, "That's the way I feel about Ric's life right now. It's rushing by, out of control. Only occasionally do I recognize a familiar part of the wonderful life that he had. What is going to happen to him? To us?"

Ric was arrested at 2 a.m. on August 21, 1990. We did not know what to do, or how to help. We just sat together, held each other and wept retching sobs. The three year old, Jake was with us, but he was asleep. We knew we couldn't do anything until morning, we weren't even able to get any information from authorities as to what had happened.

Just a week ago, I found (in one of my famous spiral notebooks) this prayer my broken heart had written. It was dated, August 21, 1990-5am. I had tearfully read it to James at that time, and he agreed this was his prayer as well.

Dear God,

I do not know why we are going through these difficult times.

Lord, if it is for cleansing our hearts and lives, we yield to Thee and ask that this be accomplished.

If it is to remind us that we are totally dependent on you, we truly acknowledge this.

If it is for us to feel your presence and care in a new and different way, we thank you for it.

Lord, if it is for us to trust you more, we do.

If it is for us to recognize again that thou art all powerful and in control of our lives and our children's, we thank Thee.

But, oh dear God, if it is for us to remember that "Our God is able to do exceeding abundantly above all that we ask or think,"

If it is for us and others to see a great miracle, we will be eternally grateful.

You know our hearts are so heavy, we are so afraid, we're tired and we're weary.

We praise you Father and thank you for what you are going to do.

Lord, please help us as a family to be kind, loving and gentle with one another.

Encouraging and uplifting each other.

Thank you for your sustaining grace and mercy and for your answered prayers.

We love you, Lord."

I share this part, because one of the greatest heartaches of parents, is seeing unfulfilled dreams crumble senselessly concerning their children. Regardless of the circumstances it is hard. But there is hope!

Hope and even answered prayers do not always come immediately. Our son went through many more difficult times, and so did we.

Ric went from jail into a wonderful Drug and Alcohol Rehab Program at Charter by the Sea, on St. Simons Island, Ga. His life was good for two years. Then he started back on drugs.

Ric was always a sweet son to us, a loving father to Jake and a wonderful, helpful brother to Melany. He was kind and considerate to all.

Addiction has its own demons. It has a way of negating many good things in all the lives it affects.

In 1993 Ric went to Hebron Colony in Boone, N.C. for a twelve week program. This is a faith based program, and a wonderful one. Also, it is free, but they have work responsibilities while there. His life (and all of ours) was great for two more years.

In 1995 he was back on drugs. It was devastating to him and us as well. He went back to Hebron. Ric's testimony was that the first time the program got into his head, the second time it really got into his heart.

Life was wonderful, once again. We all learned just to enjoy and appreciate the good times. He was working, actively involved in church and enjoying life with family and friends.

In October 1997 Ric was working in Richmond, Va. I told in Chapter IX of his visiting Melany in the hospital when she was so ill. Actually, he visited just about every week-end that he could. Two weeks before his last visit, he had shared several things with Melany. He said, "I know that Mother and Dad are concerned about me being so far away and daily battling my problems with drugs. But really, I am doing well." He continued, "Baby, I had rather be dead, than living like I have in the past because of my addiction." I have thought of this many times since his death.

Thankfully, we had those last good times to remember. Ric was killed October 23, 1997. Regardless of the drug situation and all of the heartaches and disappointments that it caused, we were thankful that he had enjoyed his last years on earth, and that God had allowed us to share them with him. Our faith, and belief according to the scriptures is that Ric is in Heaven.

I know with certainty by his testimony that he accepted Christ as his Savior when he was young. He prayed the sinner's prayer, confessed his sin of unbelief and was sealed by the Holy Spirit for eternity. He acknowledged that he had often moved away from Christ, but Christ never moved away from him. He rededicated his heart and life to the Lord when he was at Hebron the last time. Thus his renewed fellowship with Christ brought him much happiness.

The scripture attests to this, our beliefs in John 10:27-30-- Jesus' own words were:

"My sheep hear my voice, and I know them, and they follow me;
And I give unto them eternal life, and they shall never perish,
Neither shall any man pluck them out of my hand.
My Father, which gave them to me, is greater than all;
And no man is able to pluck them out of my Father's hand.
I and my father are one."

When we accept Christ, we are sealed by the Holy Spirit.
"And grieve not the Holy Spirit of God, whereby Ye are sealed unto the day of redemption." Ephesians 4:30.

What assurance and comfort to all believers.

I'm sure that Ric is enjoying his Lord, his dad, and his sisters, and just waiting for the rest of us to get there.

Finally, I understood part of God's purpose in allowing him to go through all of these hard times.

Several of his former friends came and said that they had accepted the Lord, because of seeing how happy Ric was when his life was really changed. Five of those young people, Joe, Sharon, Tommie, Danny and Mike have since died. His death had forced them to face the possible brevity of their own life. I gave the tape of Ric's funeral to a friend of his, who passed it around. John Bryan and Sherrell Dunn had presented the plan of salvation and told of God's grace to change lives, so beautifully, yet profoundly. Several friends had responded to the message, and came to us for help. The Sovereignty of God always works, we just don't always realize it at the time. We may not live to see it happen, but it does. That is how we should handle all of life, in faith and trust of our Heavenly Father, who makes no mistakes.

I had placed a poem in James' Funeral Program. It was one that we read often during the "dark" days that Ric was deep in addiction. It reminded us that only God can really give us comfort and that He can give us "songs in the night."

BEEN THROUGH THE VALLEY

"I have been through the valley of weeping,
The valley of sorrow and pain;
But the 'God of of all comfort' was with me,
At hand to uphold and sustain.

As the earth needs the clouds and sunshine,
Our souls need both sorrow and joy;
So He places us oft in the furnace,
The dross from the gold to destroy.

When He leads thro' some valley of trouble,
His omnipotent hand we trace;
For the trials and sorrows He sends us,
Are part of His lessons in grace.

Oft we shrink from the purging and pruning,
Forgetting the Husbandman knows
That the deeper the cutting and paring,
The richer the cluster that grows.

Well He knows that affliction is needed;
He has a wise purpose in view,
And in the dark valley He whispers,
"Hereafter Thou'lt know what I do."

As we travel thro' life's shadow'd valley,
Fresh springs of His love ever rise;
And we learn that our sorrows and losses,
Are blessings just sent in disguise.

So we'll follow wherever He leadeth,
Let the path be dreary or bright;
For we've proved that our God can give comfort;
Our God can give songs in the night."

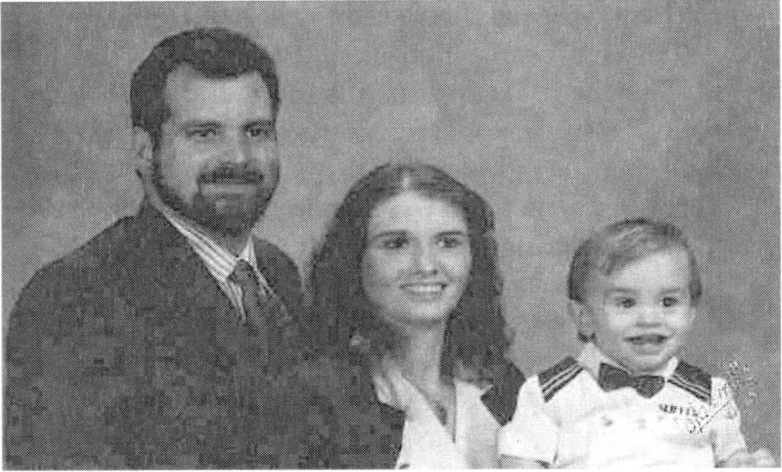

Ric with wife Charlotte and Jake

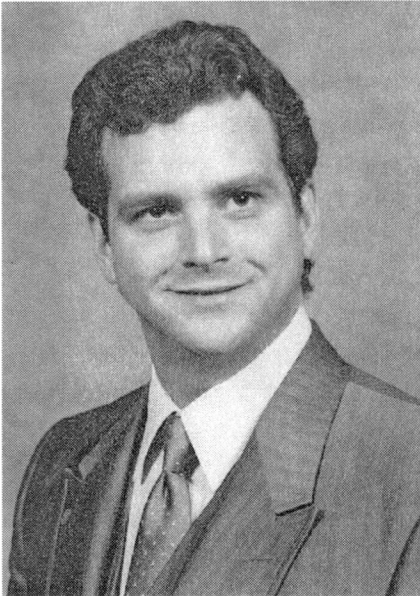

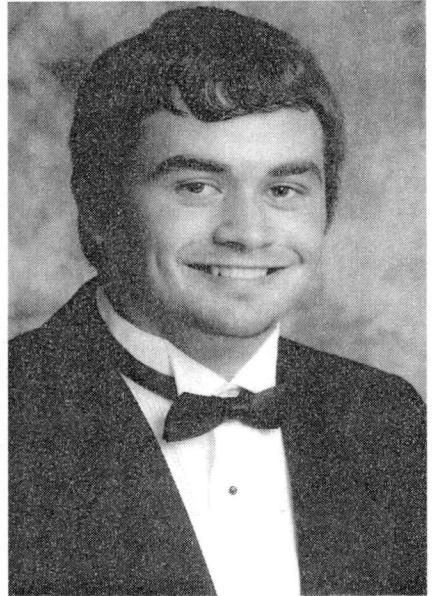

Ric (left) as adult; Jake (right) looks like his dad

In <u>Finding Hope When Life Is Not Fair</u>,
Thomas Moore reminds us that,

"Earth has no sorrow that Heaven cannot heal."

The time to trust
Is in this moment's need,
Poor, broken, bruised reed!
Poor troubled soul, make speed,
To trust thy God.

The time to trust
Is when our joy is fled,
When sorrow bows the head.
And all is cold and dead,
All else but God!
SELECTED
STREAMS IN THE DESERT

CHAPTER XVII
PEACE AND CONTENTMENT

"Lord, there is none beside thee to help."
II Chronicles 14:11 (RV)

"Be still amd know that I am God."
Psalm 46:10

After Melany's funeral, I stayed in her condo, where I had been for quite some time. Jake stayed in my other condos. I had never lived alone before. I had gone from my parents' home, straight to mine and James' new life together. I wasn't sure that I knew how to live alone or survive, but I knew that I wanted to let Jake live his own life.

I started trying to adjust to my new life. I, who had only wanted to be a wife and mother all of my life, suddenly realized I was neither. I didn't know who I was. I had no one to think about but myself. This, I didn't know how to do. I didn't like it. I cried freely; tears are cleansing. I had been a lay counselor for many years. Although I had not done much counseling during the last five years, I had conducted classes and seminars on grief. I knew the process, I knew what to do, I just didn't seem to know how to do it now.

I counseled myself, as I had done with others. I tried to go on doing the things that were routine, I read my Bible every day, and found great comfort as usual in God's Word. Although, some days I just couldn't concentrate. I did not try to get into any deep studies, I just read. I fed the birds, watered the plants every morning and evening. I watched the sunsets over the lake every evening, just as James and Melany and I had always done.

I cried every day, I felt so alone.

I was mentally, physically, and emotionally exhausted. I slept a lot. One week after Melany died, I had a TIA, my blood pressure dropped dangerously low. My blood work was all messed up. My doctor said that I was one of the most physically exhausted people she had seen, and that I needed to be in the hospital for complete checking and rest. Instead, I went home and rested.

I missed my husband and children so very much. I wrote a poem about giving my last child to the Lord. At Melany's funeral service, I was able to say a few words of thanks to all. I concluded by saying from my heart,

"The Lord giveth, the Lord taketh away--
Blessed be the name of our wonderful Lord."

I was sincere before the Lord, but I did not know how difficult giving her up was going to be. I'm not a poetry writer, but I wrote the following:

SUMMER
Came with long days of light
My child was a bed.
FALL
Came with leaves so bright
My child was abed.

WINTER
Came with snowy spread
My child was abed.

SPRING
Did not come
My child was dead.

[But the joy of Spring is deep in my heart;
It will one day return even though we are apart].

I continued counseling myself, as I continued doing the routine things, I prayed every morning that the Lord would help me to keep my heart tender (never bitter), and my spirit kind (always being aware of the needs of others).

I also asked Him to help me always keep a thankful heart. I have a little plaque hanging over my coffee pot, so I will see it every day. I read it first thing every morning. It says:

"Lord, I thank you that you have given me another day to marvel and give thanks for your marvelous creations. I add, and to thank you for my blessings, and to praise you."

This starts my day right.

I have always had a thankful heart. I would list the many things that I have to be thankful for (I still do this). I am so thankful that I do not have some of the financial problems that many widows have, I have a nice home and a nice car. I have many friends (in my church, and otherwise) to check on me daily, and will help me at any time. I have a loving family. I am so thankful that all of my immediate family accepted Christ as their Savior, and that we will be together for eternity. Still I would cry out to God, "Lord, I have so much to be grateful for, but I miss my family, I hurt so badly."

Bereaved parents have several sayings, my favorite being, "You're not going crazy, you're only grieving." At times, I wondered about my sanity, I just couldn't seem to keep up with things. I couldn't remember things. Also, I did some pretty weird things. I knew this would get better at some time. I found one of their sayings to be so very true, it says: "A crowd can seem so lonely, when only one person is missing."

I went back to church and the activities that I had not been able to be a part of for a long time. I knew that many times couple friends do not include widows in their plans of going out and just getting together. I was very grateful that I was still included. Weekly (sometimes more often), I was invited to go with them. I would cry as they left together, and I had to go home alone. I never let them know this, I didn't want them to feel badly. I did find later in my "healing" that I found it was better for me, and probably for them too if I limited these times.

I was finding that being a widow brought many surprises and often confusion, as well as the expected pain. I was surprised at the pain the first time I had to check "widow" at a doctor's office. I realized, this is final, but I don't want to be a widow!

I was surprised that I handled some things that I dreaded doing, so well; and yet I fell apart at little things, such as a song, seeing a white Cadillac Eldorado like James drove. I see one often, and I tear up every time.

To this day, My heart still cries when I go by the little girl's dresses in a store, or see a beautiful little girl and a mother together. Also, when I see the little boys suited up in their uniforms of any kind, for their sports events. I have the same feelings when I see an elderly couple together, fortunate enough "to grow old together."

I knew several things about grief for certain:

> You cannot stop it,
> You cannot side-step it,
> You cannot ignore it,
> You cannot avoid it,
> You have to walk through it--all the way,
> One step at a time,
> Every painful step.

Otherwise you will not come out of it healthy; mentally, physically, emotionally or spiritually. You will get through it, it just takes some longer than others. We must be kind to ourselves and to others that do not understand.

This was sent to me, it expressed my desires exactly. I have sent it to many grieving friends.

PLEASE BE GENTLE

> *Please be gentle with me for I am grieving,*
> *The sea I swim in is a lonely one,*
> *and the shore seems miles away.*

Waves of despair numb my soul
as I struggle through each day.

My heart is heavy with sorrow, I want to
shout and scream and repeatedly ask, "Why?"
At times my grief overwhelms me, and I weep bitterly,
So great is my loss.

Please don't turn away or tell me to move
On with my life,
I must embrace my pain before I can begin to heal.
Companion me through my tears and sit with me
in loving silence.
Honor where I am in my journey, not where
You think I should be.

Listen patiently to my story.
I need to tell it over and over again.
It's how I begin to grasp the enormity of my loss.
Nurture me through the weeks and months ahead.

Forgive me when I seem distant and inconsolable.
A small flame still burns within my heart,
And shared memories may trigger both
Laughter and tears.
I need your support and understanding.

There is no right or wrong way to grieve.
I must find my own path.
Please, will you walk beside me?
Carol Adams

I found I was quite content as long as I stayed at home.
When I left my home, even for a little while, I dreaded coming
home and going in alone. I disciplined myself to only cry the
first thing every morning, as I looked at the pictures of my
precious family, and the last thing at night. Of course, I did cry

unexpectedly sometime, however I tried to not make others uncomfortable.

A real surprise came on July 24, my fifty-third wedding anniversary. I had thought about the approaching day for several days. James and I had done that for several years. We enjoyed remembering how young and inexperienced we were, and some of the funny things that preceded our wedding. I went to bed the night before enjoying these sweet memories. When I awoke the next morning, I had an overwhelming need for my husband. It really surprised me, and I thought it would go away, but it didn't. I discreetly tried talking to some friends who were widowed. They seemed to think that I was ridiculous to have such thoughts at my age. I really felt alone, there must be something bad wrong with me, maybe I was losing my mind. A dear pastor friend helped me to see that it was intimacy that I craved. James and I had enjoyed a very nurturing relationship, and I was missing that. I realized then, how much I really missed the physical touch of my mate. I share this here, because I have since heard several widows express similar feelings (usually younger ones), and they could not find anyone to talk to about it, everyone seems to avoid this issue. It is very real, at any age. It is very painful, it is now being addressed in several grief programs, as it should be.

*   *   *   *

A couple of weeks before my anniversary, Jake and I had attended our shareholders meeting for the company that James and his cousins had founded. They had planned a meaningful Memorial Service for James and had a beautiful portrait of him there. Many people said many endearing things about him. They had asked me to say a few words, which I gladly did.

It was a bittersweet time. Jake and I stayed down for the Powell (James' mother's family) Reunion on Sunday. We stayed in Vidalia until the next Saturday and attended the Wiggins reunion. It was all very enjoyable.

I knew that I had to build a different life, I just didn't know how. I knew also, that I could and should take my time doing it.

I was aware I had lived a very happy fulfilled life. I was beginning to acknowledge just how involved I had been with the needs and desires of my family. While having dinner one evening with several couple friends, I was asked what my favorite television programs were. I realized and shared with them, that I didn't have any. I just always watched whatever James or Melany wanted to watch. They all laughed, but I was serious. So, I started trying to watch some programs. I did not watch the programs that I had shared with them, it was to painful, and I really didn't care for some of the programs that they watched. I have found a few that I like, but I really am not an avid watcher. I do enjoy some movies, if they have a happy ending.

I started trying to do some positive things, they included:
1- Continuing going to church and activities.
2- Going to our Labor Day get together at the lake.
3- Visiting Roger and Rosa at their mountain home.
4- Attending my family reunion in South Georgia.
5- Visiting family in Charlotte, N.C.
6- Attending a Senior Conference at Toccoa, GA.
7- Started attending Bereaved Parents Meetings.
8- Going to a Grief Share Program.

Many of these things were quite enjoyable, some sad, others painful and some bittersweet. I still had time to revisit many happy times in our lives. But I also allowed my grief process to continue at its own pace.

In November, I attended a "Grief Share for the Holidays," and a similar session in "Bereaved Parents." Both had many good suggestions. Such as changing the way you have celebrated, going away for the holidays, trying to not overdo or overstress yourself. Remembering that other family members and friends were suffering too. As many shared their own ways of celebrating, many were choosing not to. As I said earlier, there is no right or wrong way to handle grief and pain.

I had never even thought of not celebrating Thanksgiving or

Christmas. I decorated my house for the fall and Thanksgiving, and found comfort in doing so. Of course, I had my "moments."

Both groups had memorial services for our loved ones. Many family members and friends attended. Many thoughts were shared and many tears were shed.

I chose to attend all of the Christmas Programs and Services that I could, crying through many of them. They were all so beautiful and meaningful.

I had started decorating for Christmas the day after Thanksgiving. I cried constantly as I hung the meaningful ornaments on the tree. I still have all the little things that my children made through the years. Each year, we had given them an inexpensive shiny ornament with their name and the year engraved on it.

This year we would celebrate Christmas in a different but a special way. Jake's mother, Charlotte was coming from Florida, and Frannie (Jake's half sister) and Jeremy and their two boys were coming from Hartsville, S.C. I still had many times of sitting alone enjoying the lights of the Christmas Trees, and taking a journey back to past times shared.

I still have a Christmas Tree in each room, including the bathrooms. I have a large one in my living room and a fifty year old silver tree with blue balls that was my mothers. A beautiful ceramic tree that my mother-in-law made has a special place in my living room, as well as in my heart. Many joys remembered, many tears freely shed.

I wrote the following poem that a friend later gave to the local newspaper. It was later printed in two monthly papers as well.

CHRISTMAS CELEBRATION

It's the weeks before Christmas
When all through the room--
Sweet memories are stirring
Without any gloom.

The house is all decorated
The trees brightly lit--
My family members are all gone
And now alone I sit.

I think of wonderful
Christmas' past--
Knowing life's fragile treasures
Do not forever last.

Alone, but not lonely
Christ is with me always--

And it's really His birth
I celebrate these days!

Christmas Eve and Christmas Day was very different, but enjoyable. It was fun watching the great-grandchildren on Christmas morning.

After lunch we invited the four neighborhood children to join our children and we gathered in our front yard. I had purchased some helium-inflated balloons, as I had done for Jake for Christmas after Ric died eleven years ago. Charolotte and Frannie had written the children's names on the balloons with magic markers. They had also written "Papa" on one and "Melany" on another. Happy Birthday Jesus was written on the fourth one. We had four for each child. However, we only gave them one at a time.

First they released the one with their name on it, then Papa's, followed by Melany's. Each time they shouted "Miss you Papa," then "Miss you Mimi."

We had a simple brief prayer, thanking God for our family and for Jesus. Then they each let the final one go Heavenward as they sang Happy Birthday to Jesus. They all "squealed" with glee as they watched them all go up into the sky and finally out of sight. They each insisted that they could still see the one with their name on it.

We repeated this the next year, and many neighbors joined us. The children still remember it and talk about the experience.

On January 30, 2009, Melany's group of friends all came to celebrate her forty-second birthday. They had asked ahead of time if they could come. Of course, I said yes. They brought all the food. Stan brought the birthday cake. They each shared something funny that they remembered about Melany, then they shared some other thoughts. It was a great night. It was another one of those bittersweet times.

On February 4, I placed a one year memorial picture of James and a poem in the local newspaper. It was the poem that James had shared with me in 2007, about when he was gone. Many called and said that it meant a lot to them, and caused them to be very thoughtful about the message of going on with life. I really was trying! Some days I felt I did good, some not so good.

I had started typing Melany's Book, as I had promised her I would do. It was very emotional. The first chapters of "Prittle" and "Prattle" were fun to review and type. But from "Pain" on, it became more and more difficult.

The typewriter that I had was obsolete and beyond repair. I had to learn to type on the computer, which I had avoided for a long time. It took me a long time to type and not accidentally erase it. Jake was very patient with me, most of the time. I don't think that he believed that I could be so dumb, and such a slow learner. I did get better, with a lot of practice.

When Melany had dictated the thoughts and words to me, as I wrote them in the large spiral notebook I had simply abbreviated some and spelled some of them as I thought they were, or as they sounded. I didn't want to break her concentration, by stopping her to spell the words. I thought that we would correct them when I typed, never knowing it would be so long, and that I would have to do alone,

I was in quite a dilemma. I called Melany's Dr. Magruder, who was retired. I asked him about some medical words and phrases and how to spell them. He so graciously offered to come over and help me. I was so grateful, he offered just the help that I needed so badly. We became very good friends.

In looking back, it is overwhelming what all he has done for me. He had lost his dear wife, Carolyn one month before James's death. He was James' doctor for twenty years, as well as Melany's for thirty years. He had sent me nice cards with caring messages after they both died.

I had always greatly admired him through the years, and my admiration of him increased. He just seemed to handle everything in his life so easily. Certainly I'm sure everything in his life had not and did not always run smoothly, but he never seemed to get upset about it.

I had known his wife through the times that she worked in the office with him, as I had to take Melany there often. I had always admired her. She was a lovely, talented lady and I know he loved her dearly. I'm sure he grieved deeply, but he seemed to adjust so well. Especially compared to my life that just seemed completely unraveled.

I often felt like a ship without a rudder, just drifting in a big lake. Occasionally I'd drift into a small cove, where I felt comfortable and safe. Then I would drift aimlessly back into the big waters, with no direction or idea of where I was going. I didn't know where to go next, or what to do.

Richard helped me considerably, not with just the medical things, but with getting my life back on track. One thing that he did regularly was to go to our local Family Y everyday and exercise. He suggested that I go and do the water exercises.

I have never liked to exercise, because I don't like pain and I hate to sweat. Getting into the water appealed to me. I had always loved to swim, and I hadn't done that for years. So I enrolled, and started going three to five days a week. It has been great for my health and very enjoyable!

In I Timothy 5:13 the Bible warns the young widows (I'm sure this applies to older widows as well) about "being idle, wandering about from house to house; and not only being idle, but tattlers also and busybodies, speaking things which they ought not." I certainly wanted to avoid this.

We need time for thinking, planning and formulating how to get our lives back in order. But it's obvious Paul knew we widows didn't need too much idle time on our hands or we could get into lots of trouble.

I continued trying to do normal things:

Reading my Bible and praying.

Watering my flowers morning and evening.

Feeding the birds.

Watching sunsets.

One evening I was so sad. I cried out, "Lord, I am so lonely, couldn't you have left at least one of them for a little while longer?" He said so clearly to my heart and mind, "Which one would you have chosen to keep?" I answered, "Oh Lord, I'm so glad that I never had to make that choice. You know what is best for me. I want you to always be in charge of my life and my actions."

In Streams In The Desert, J.H. McC. Writes,

"Friend, you do not have to understand all God's ways with you. God does not expect you to understand them. You do not expect your child to understand, only believe. Some day you will see the glory of God in the things which you do not understand."

I made several trips, continued visiting friends and family. I went back to Toccoa. Then I went on a wonderful cruise with family members.

I spent two weeks at St. Simons. It was very hard to go back there without James and Melany. It was nice to see so many friends, they entertained me constantly, and I truly enjoyed the beach, our church, and the relaxed life on the island.

I continued having surprises. I was surprised that I still had a hard time seeing couples together, even my close friends. I really prayed about this. I had never had any jealousy or envy in my life, I surely didn't want to start now. I wasn't sure what I was feeling. The Lord did help me to identify that I was going through a normal adjustment. I did find it more comfortable when I stopped going out so often with couple friends. I'm sure some of them was secretly glad that they did not have to look at me (and often my pain), and face the brevity of their own time together. I continued going out with my girl friends regularly.

I was also surprised that instead of longing for Heaven to see and be with Jesus, as I had always done, I longed to see and be with James, and my children more. I felt that this was wrong. Mark Harris helped me to see that it was alright at this time. That Jesus understood our feelings in times like this. He said just stay in the Word, and you will be alright. He was right.

Another surprise that I had was that I started "dating" or whatever you call it when people my age go out for dinner. The first couple of times, I still had on my wedding and engagement rings. Then a friend told me that I should take them off. I hadn't thought of that, I knew I had a lot to learn.

Ten guys asked me out several times, and it was enjoyable. Two actually asked me to marry them, that surprised me too, I hadn't thought about marrying again.

My widowed friends were quite surprised also, and some of them expressed it to me, asking why I was asked out and they weren't. I certainly didn't know either. I suppose I am average looking for a mature lady, in her seventies. But I'm certainly nothing special. Several of them are beautiful and special. I told them I thought it was apparently the year of "Be kind to old ladies in wheelchairs." These nice men were getting older and they were probably trying to make points with the Lord. I was just as amazed as they were!

Going out was fun for a while, but I soon got tired of this. I wanted a relationship, but not now. I had a lot of work I needed to be doing. I recognized my life was not ready to get involved with a relationship. I just asked God, if it was his will for this to happen, then I trusted Him to bring it about, and help me to be ready for it.

*   *   *   *

I missed my family so much, at times it was almost unbearable. I have used the devotional book <u>Streams In The Desert,</u> by Mrs. Charles Cowman since 1997. I have had much comfort in the years from this devotional book. So, again I found just the words I needed to hear.

"Be strong my soul!

Thy loved ones go

Within the veil, God's thine, even so;

Be strong.

Be strong, my soul!

Death looms in view.

Lo, hear thy God! He'll bear thee through;

Be strong."

"Storms of bereavement are keen; but, then, they are one of the Father's ways of driving me to Himself, that in the secret of His presence His voice may speak to my heart, soft and low."

It was as though the following poem was sent directly to me from our loving Heavenly Father.

"My peace I give when thou art left alone--

The nightingale at night has sweetest tone.

My peace I give in time of utter loss,

The way of glory leads right to the cross.

My peace I give when there's but death for thee

The gateway is the cross to get to me." L.S.P.

On May thirteenth, Melany's death date, we had a picture of Melany in the memorial section of our paper with a poem that she loved and had asked to have in her order of service for her funeral. I couldn't find it at that time. It was her sentiments exactly, and I did want to share it.

I'M FREE

Don't grieve for me, for now I'm free,
I'm following the path God laid for me.
I took His hand when I heard Him call,
I turned my back and left it all.

I could not stay another day,
To laugh, to love, to work or play.
Tasks left undone must stay that way,
I found that place at the close of the day.

If my passing has left a void,
Then fill it with remembered joy
A friendship shared, a laugh, a kiss,
Ah yes, these things, I too, will miss.
Be not burdened with times of sorrow,
I wish for you the sunshine of tomorrow.
My life's been full, I savored much,
Good friends, good times, a loved one's touch.

Perhaps my time seemed all too brief,
Don't lengthen it now with undue grief.
Lift up your heart and share with me,
God wanted me now, He set me free.

Jo Lynn Jackson

"O how blessed is the promise
When our spirit is set free;
To be absent from the body,
Means to live, O Lord, with Thee!"
(Bosch)

Surprises continued, some that I did not understand. I feel three and one half years after James' death, that my journey of grief is where it should be. I miss him, but acute grief seems gone. I know memories will always stay, and a certain amount of pain will remain.

The surprise is that I have not yet gotten my grief over Melany in the proper perspective. I have thought much about this. I miss all of my children, but I had Melany with me the longest. This may be part of it.

I guess the Lord spared me some of grief, by allowing James to go to Canada for long periods of time, and only come home most weekends. Then for the last four years he was in Vidalia, and only home for the weekends. So I do not mentally expect him to come home every day at the same time, like most husbands do.

Melany and I were together almost constantly for the last five years of her life. I stayed in her condo with her during the week while James was gone. So when I leave now, and return to the home that I shared with Melany, I miss her so much.

I believe that perhaps the real reason that I am not handling grief over Melany as well as I have handled my other times of grief, is because I don't have James to depend on and to share my grief.

As I think back to the Christmas Eve that I lost our first baby, who was stillborn, I remember James just encircling me in his arms, and holding me for long periods of time as I wept uncontrollably. He would repeat, "It's going to be OK." After a long time, it was. When the other two deaths occurred, he did the same thing. I felt that when he held me, everything would be alright. Now as I deal with Melany's death, I do not have this comfort. But I know that God is a great comforter in time of need. I will get through this grief, it just may take me a little longer.

*   *   *   *   *

In January 2009, Jake and I started getting some calls from the shareholders stating that the business James had been involved with was having troubles. We considered the calls, and decided that most were probably just unhappy that the invention was not ready to sell, and they were anxious for their returns.

At the shareholders annual meeting in July, I gave an appeal for patience and to just trust the other partner and his decisions. I told them that James trusted him, and so did I. Things seemed better for several months.

In February 2010, more problems were being brought to our attention. Jake's help to me again became invaluable. He helped me as we started looking into the situation.

We found several things in the PPM that was not being done correctly, according to our understanding. We went down and tried to get some answers and some clarity concerning several things. The other two partners said there was nothing to worry about. We asked to see the records. They refused, even though I am third partner of the business, and we knew that any shareholder had a right to this information during normal business hours. Things became heated, we didn't insist, we just left.

We knew then, that something was definitely wrong. Jake and I consulted our attorney and a corporate lawyer. They both gave us suggestions that could hopefully get the business straightened out and again running right.

We went back six more times. They refused any help and treated us very badly. I have never had such pain in my heart or life. I felt used and betrayed by the partners.

One of the most helpless and sad feelings came because I knew that many others had been betrayed as well. James had sold shares to many family members and friends, as well as many others that had trusted him and the others. James had never been involved with any of the financial part of the business. He died thinking that things were going nicely.

I was told that I should sue the other partners on behalf of all the shareholders, or they could come after me as well. I was horrified. James did not believe in suing, certainly not a family member.

This caused me much grief and pain. I prayed and prayed about it. Then a little over a month before the next shareholders meeting in July, my devotional for June 15, was as follows.

"Bereavements are raining into my life which are making my shrinking heart quiver in its intensity of suffering. The rain of affliction is surely beating down upon my soul these days."

"You shrink from the suffering. But God sees the tender compassion for other suffers which is finding birth in your soul.

Your heart winces under the sore bereavement. But God sees the deepening and enriching which that sorrow has brought to you.

It isn't raining afflictions for you. It is raining tenderness, love, compassion, patience and a thousand others flowers and fruits of the blessed Spirit, which are bringing into your life such a spiritual enrichment as all the fullness of worldly prosperity and ease was never able to beget in your innermost soul."   J.M.McC

I felt that I had my answer. According to those that knew, and the three attorneys that we had consulted, a suit was seemingly the only way to get the attention and hopefully co-operation of the other partners, then perhaps we could move the company forward. Painfully and sorrowfully I advised our attorneys to proceed. It would come up at the shareholders meeting.

But just as often happens, when we are obedient to what we believe is the leading of the Lord, even if we don't understand it, God provided another way.

The Shareholders Meeting usually lasts two hours or less. This one lasted four and a half hours. There was much discussion, anger against the other partners became very loud and filled with exasperation. Finally, the miracle happened, the partner, being the CEO, stepped down and nominated a new one that was very acceptable to all. A new board was elected and we left on a guarded but happy note.

It didn't last long. The new board worked diligently to try to reconstruct the business. I financed all of necessary money to keep the company going. I knew that is what James would want me to do. The partner would not agree to anything that the new board wanted to do. He was still the major shareholder, holding the majority of the votes. The board even tried to approach him in the manner that is described in Matthew 15:15-17. They went individually, went by twos, then went by threes. All efforts they made were rejected.

Now one year later, we have been to court several times, and to many hearings. We have no resolution at this time. The shareholders have been very kind to Jake and me, they have been extremely patient. but they are again getting anxious. Many are believers, and our faith and trust remain in the Lord. He makes no mistakes! It has been a long battle, and it is not over yet.

All of the sicknesses and deaths that I have experienced have been very difficult. The pain and sorrow that I have had this last year ranks among my greatest sorrows.

Until this happened, with the partners I had never had anyone that I had felt was trying to hurt me and my feelings, by the things that they did and the things that they said to me and about me. I knew also that they had hurt many other innocent people, as well. I have spent hours in God's Word, and prayer. I finally decided that maybe the Lord was using this to help me fully understand some of the problems that I seek to help others deal with. I have new empathy for many situations.

Jake and I have spent much time answering emails and phone calls. At this point it grieves us that we do not have anything encouraging to report.

Losing all of the money I have invested is nothing compared to the pain of losing the love and care I had received from the partners. They are family, my heart still hurts because they have lost a lot of their material things. They seem to blame me and do not realize or acknowledge how I tried to help them make things right and avoid possible legal suits and incarceration for them.

I truly forgive these loved ones for the pain that they have caused to me and Jake. I knew that I had to get right with God, before I could really forgive them. I knew that I could not do it on my own. But if we really want to forgive completely, then God gives us the grace to do so.

We are told in Ecclesiastes 12:14 that God will judge the secrets of our hearts. So we must completely forgive with our entire heart and mind and not just our lips. Considering the brevity of time, I may soon stand before my Lord. I want my heart to be clean with no malice or spirit of unforgiveness.

I would like to believe, and to seek to understand in my own life what Job of old said, concerning his many maladies. The paraphrase is,

> *"Are not my troubles intended*
> *to deepen my character and to robe*
> *me in graces I had little of before?"*

After four years, I feel as though I am finally coming out of a fog. I believe I am close to being in the desired place with my grieving. Grief will end one day, but some pain will remain forever.

In this book, I have told many things about our family that had been shared with very few. I have exposed our hearts, pain and suffering. I have revealed our weaknesses, human thoughts, blunderings as well as our failures and fears.

I have sought to be open and honest. It pained me greatly to share some of the things that I did. It is my sincere desire that some of the things will help someone on their difficult and perhaps similar journey.

However, I sincerely pray that I have shared our hope, though weak at times, our faith, sometimes faltering, and our trust, that was always strong in our loving God.

The Scriptures, Poems and comments were selected with great care and prayer for the proper chapters.
--But also that perhaps they would touch a heart or life that needs to receive their message.

After her many losses, Rose Kennedy was to have said,
"Even the birds sing after a violent storm.
Why shouldn't people feel as free
To delight in whatever sunlight remains to them?

It has been said,
"Some hearts, like evening
primroses,
open more beautifully in the shadows of life."

May this be my legacy.

"You have been in the storms and swept by the blasts.
Have they left you--
Broken,
Weary,
Beaten in the valley.
OR
Have they lifted you to the sunlit summits of a--
Richer,
Deeper,
More abiding manhood or womanhood?
Have they left you with more sympathy and
understanding with the--
Storm-swept and
Battle scarred?"
SELECTED

OH LORD, I PRAY SO!

EPILOGUE

I recently found this hand-written paper that Melany wrote (prior to 1997, when her brother was killed, because she mentioned him). It was to be read after her death. She had left explicit instructions for her casket, her service, pallbearers and burial. Although I had not seen this when she died, most of her wishes were carried out as she wished. I feel this is sweet and awesome for all!

"I have had a very difficult and painful life, but I've also had a happy and fulfilled life. I never wanted anyone to feel sorry for me when I was alive, and sure don't want pity now. At this moment, I'm exactly where I've longed to be. If you feel anything about me now, let it be envy.

"I tried to live my life in such a way that Christ would be glorified through my infirmities. If one person came to know Jesus as Lord and Savior because of my illness, then the years of pain and suffering would have been worth it.

"I would like to take this opportunity to apologize to anyone I might have offended during my days on earth. I know that I messed up several good relationships throughout my life, but I hope that those I have wronged can find in their heart to forgive me.

"To my parents, I would like to say that I appreciate the support and love you freely gave me. I love you and I'm glad that God chose me to be your child. Your love and care shaped my character and tamed my personality and helped me to stretch my wings and fly when others thought you should have kept m in a glass box. Thank you for giving me the freedom I needed. You did the right thing as far as I was concerned.

"To Ric, I loved you very much, my dear brother. You brought me many hours of joy and gladness and I always admired your courage and determination. The Lord has great things in store for you, if you'll allow Him to lead and direct your life.

"To my precious "Woobie" Jake, Aunt Mel loved you with her whole heart and you made my life complete. Please don't ever forget me or my love for you. I'll see you again one day, but for now please…My sincere desire for you is that you will allow Christ to be both Savior and Lord of your life and that you'll use your abundance of energy to further the cause of Christ on Earth

"To Charlotte, I am glad that I will see you one day in Glory. I wasn't very patient with you at times, but I loved you very much and I'm proud of you for changing your life and your attitude, through the power of Christ. Hang in there.

"To my very special friends, I loved you all very much and I'm glad that you allowed me to share in your lives. Each of you had a very special place in my heart and I cherished your love and prayers and support very much.   All of you were an inspiration and a joy to me, and I appreciate your endless care.

"To my Doctors, I'd like to simply say "Thank You." You all worked very hard to make my life as pleasant and pain free as possible. If you learned anything from my life, I hope it was that life without Christ means nothing and death without Him, costs everything.

"Thank you to everyone who touched my life in anyway and helped me to have the best life possible. I enjoyed sharing my life with all of you, and I'm looking forward to our reunion in Heaven.

"Until then, keep striving for the mark and proclaim Jesus as Lord.

Our God Rules!
Love, Mel"

PHOTOGRAPHS

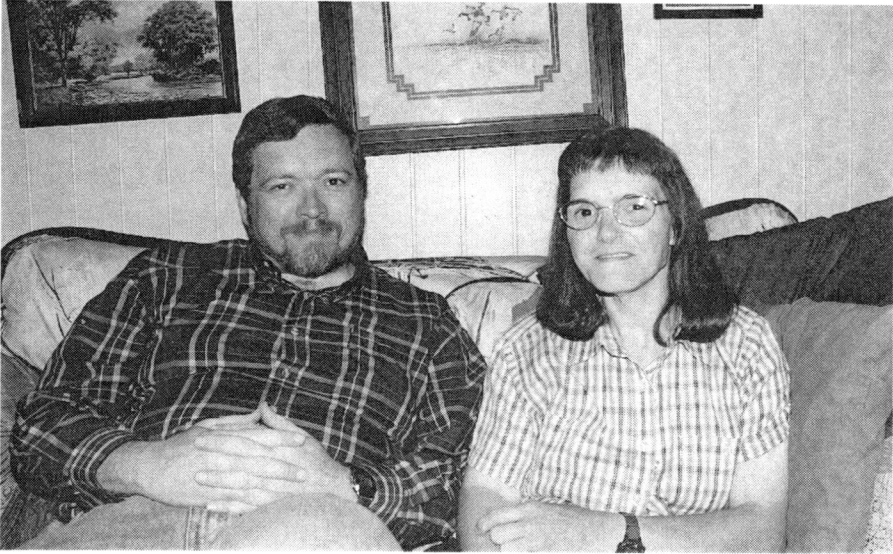

Stan Brassell with Melany

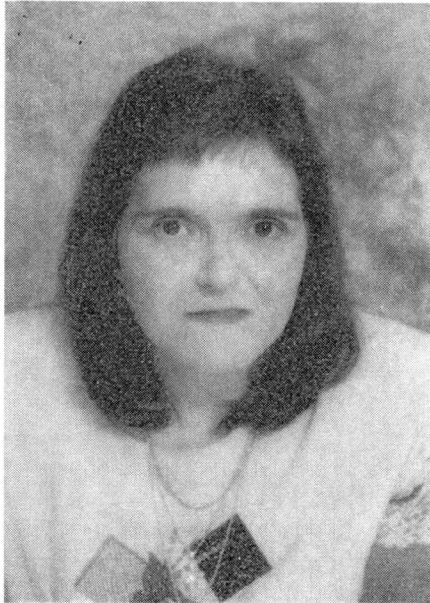

Melany in 2004

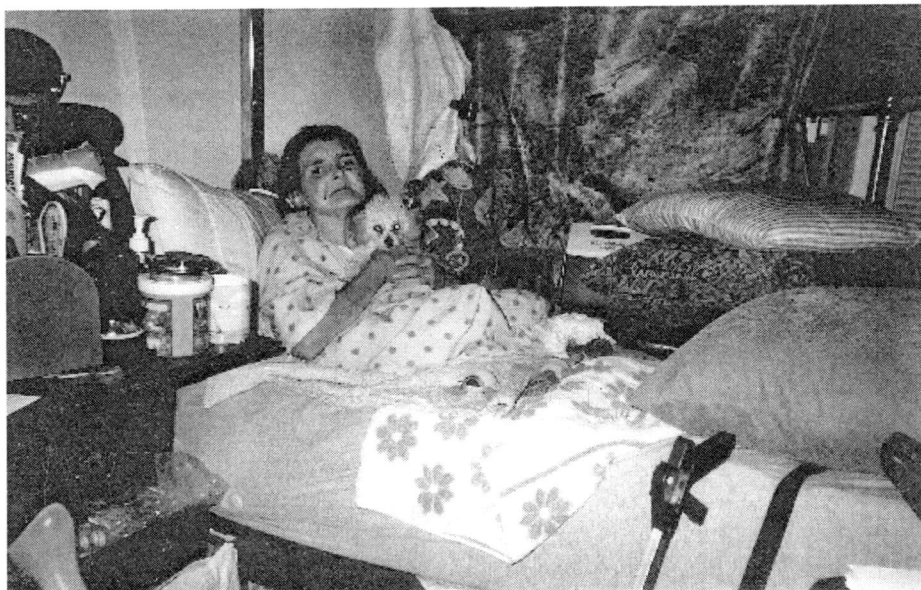

Melany in 2008

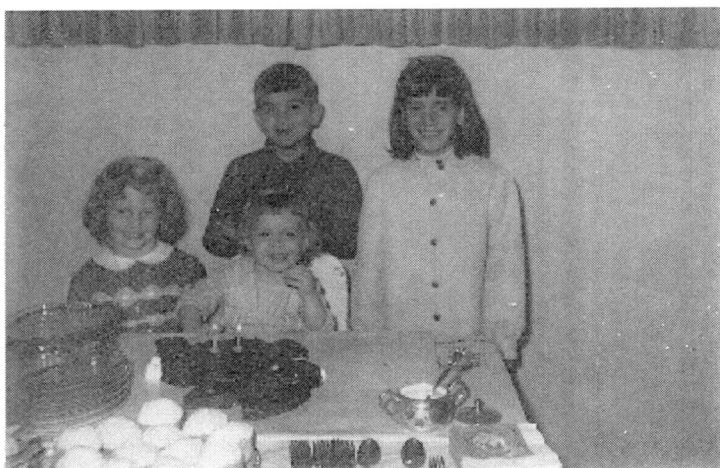

Ric, Melany, Dianne and Debbie Hudelson

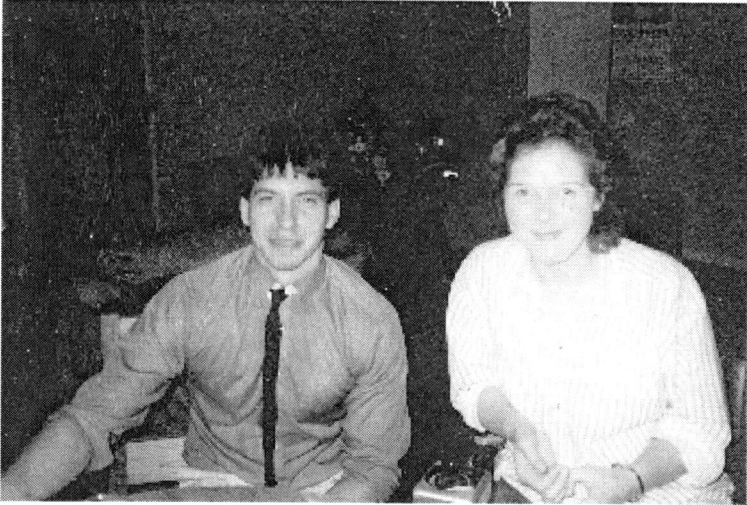

Mark and Melany

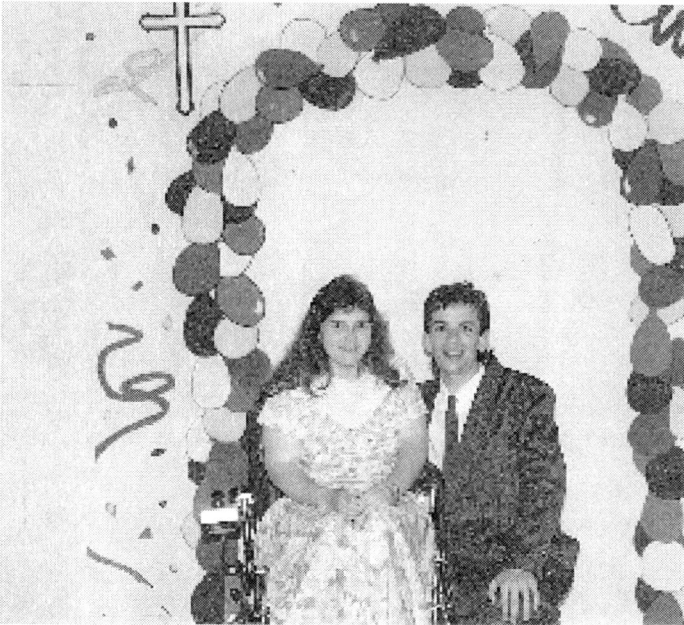

Melany and Chris

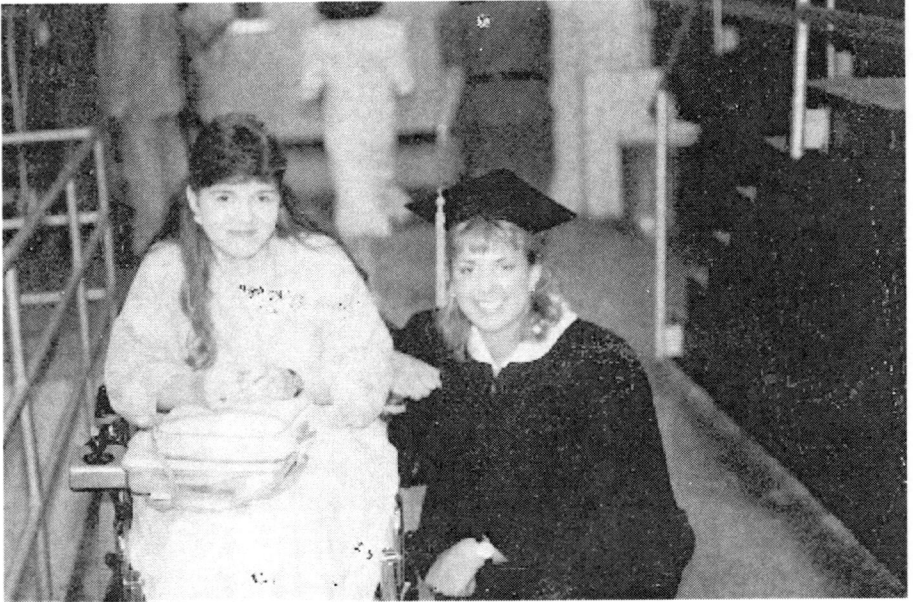

Melany and Rebecca

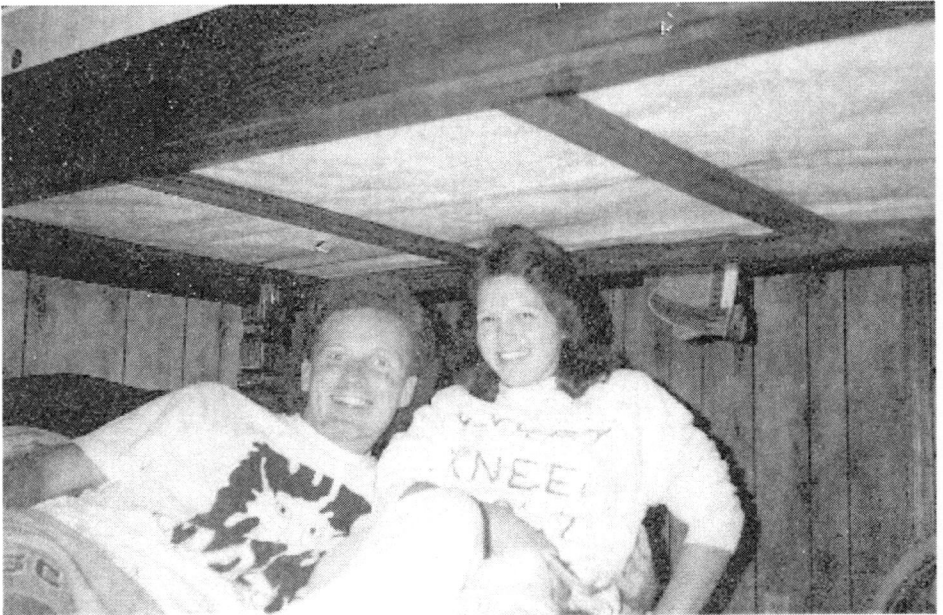

Melany and Toby

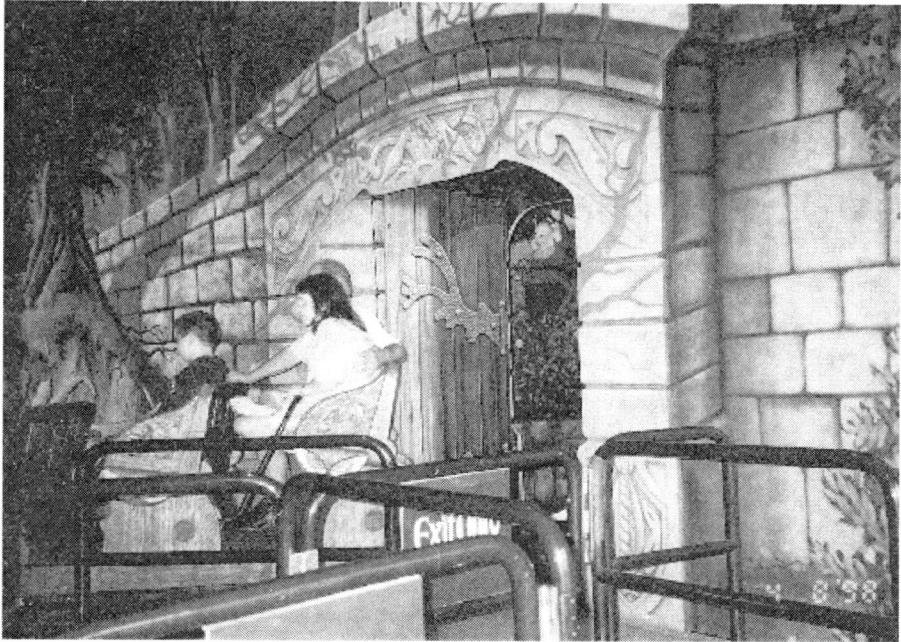
Melany with Dad and Jake at Disney World 1998

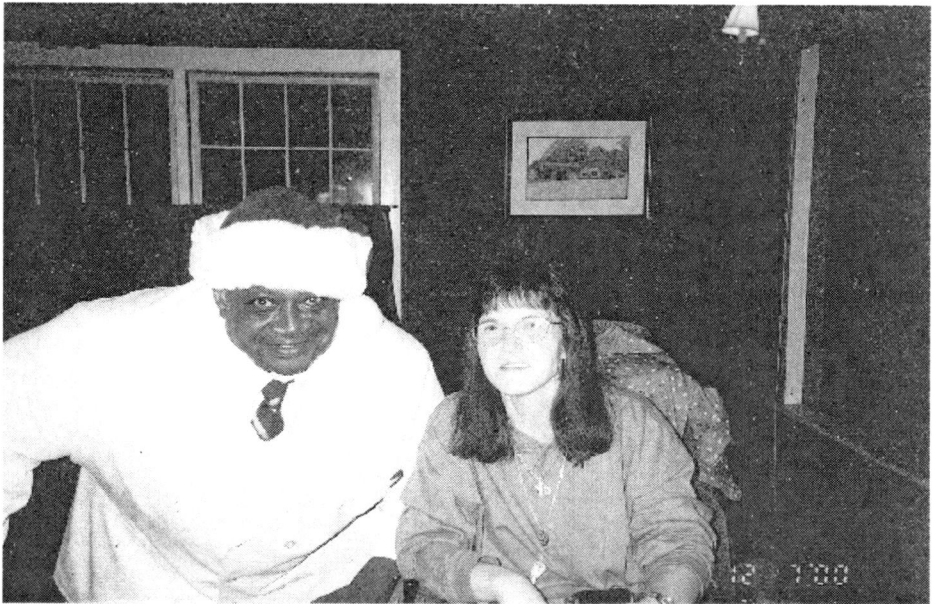
Melany and "Honored Employee"
of many years at Red Barn - St. Simons Island

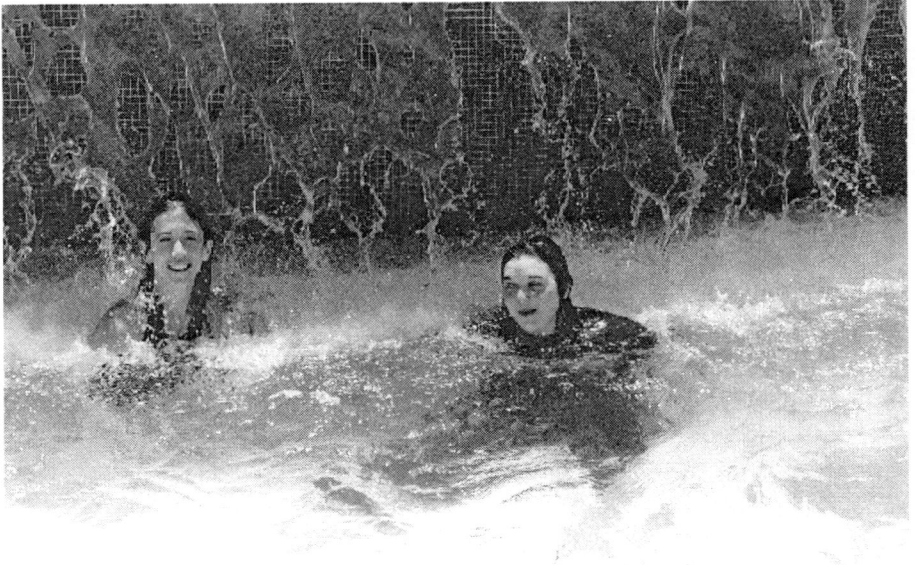

Melany and Julie in pool

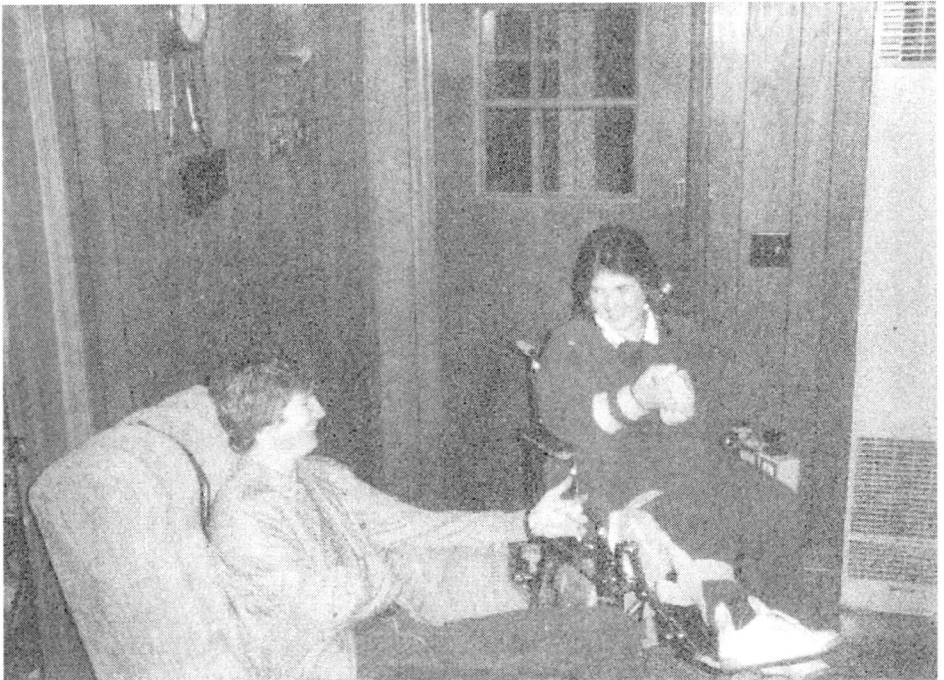

Melany and Greg

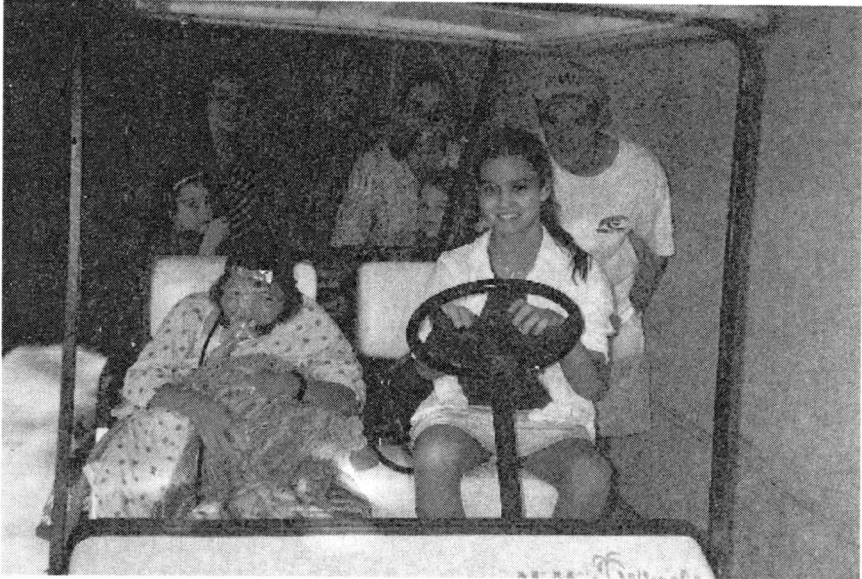
Melany, Noel and her children
(Melany's last trip to St. Simons, 2006)

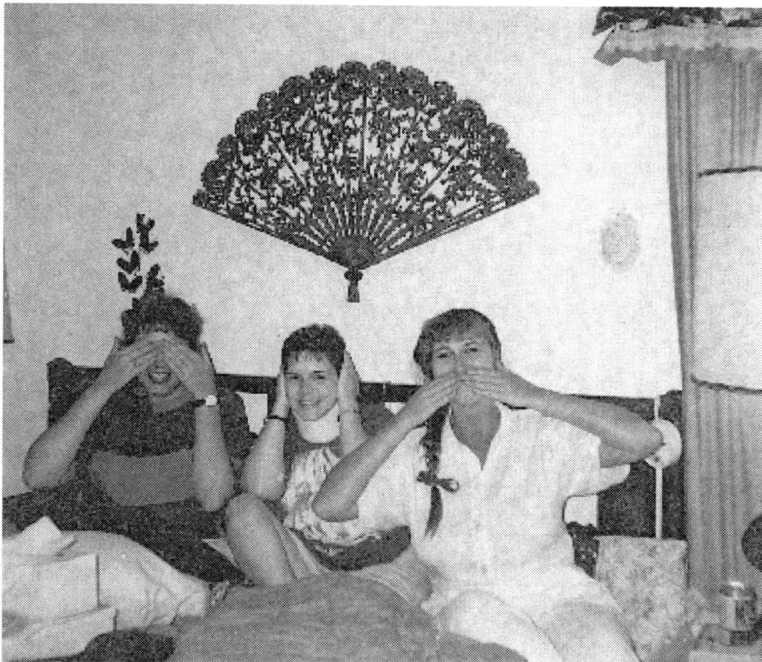
Lisa, Rebecca and Melany (see no evil, hear no evil, speak no evil)

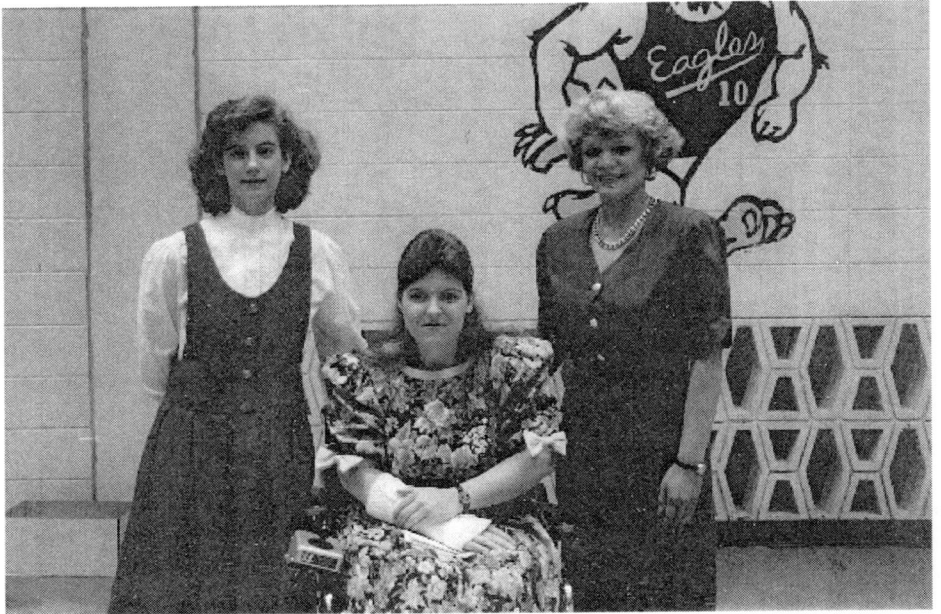

Janet, Melany and Dana

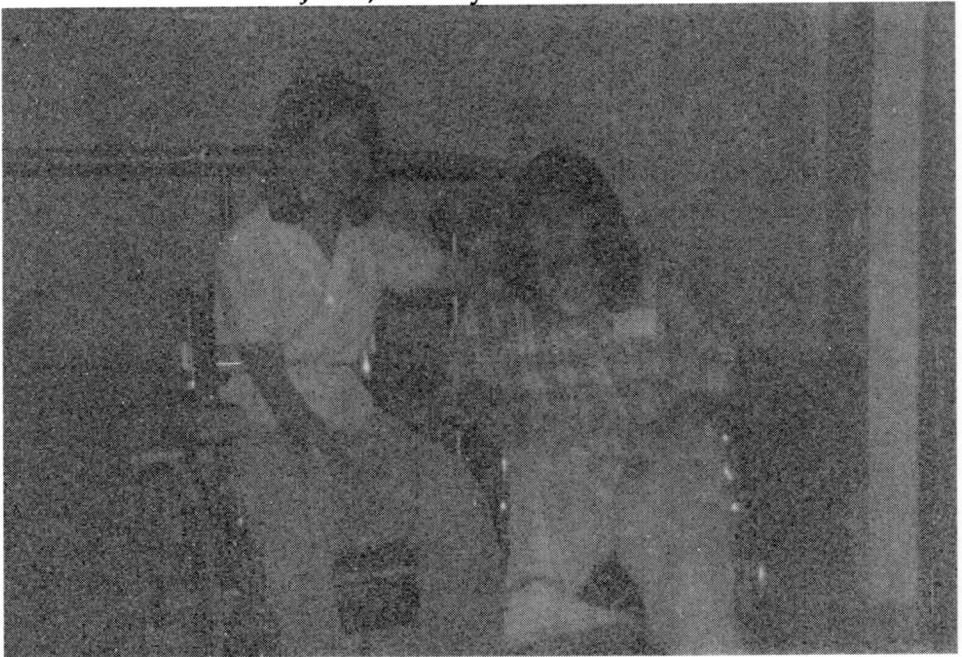

Melany and Johnie Erickson Tada

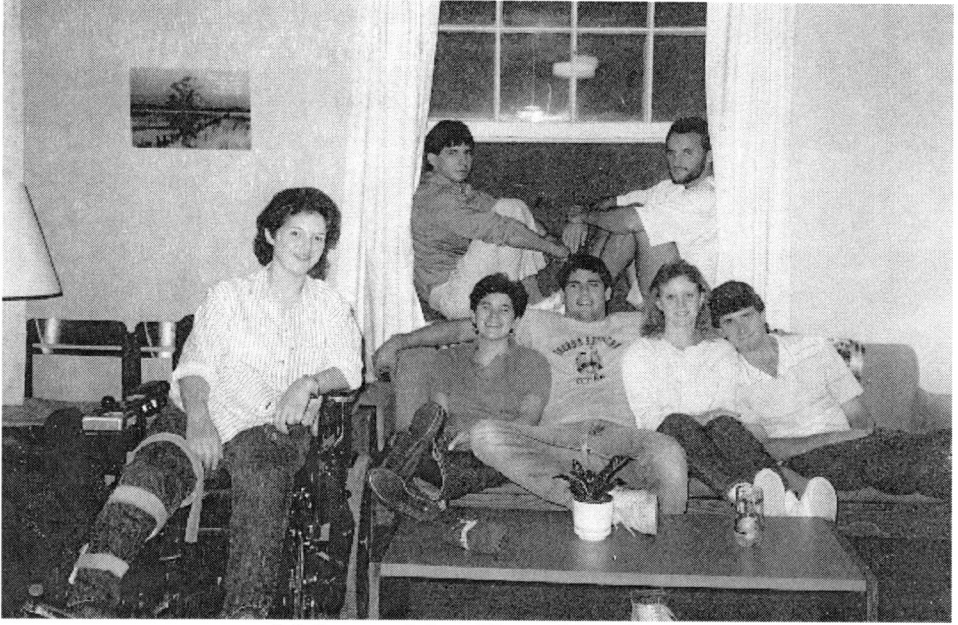
Melany with college friends

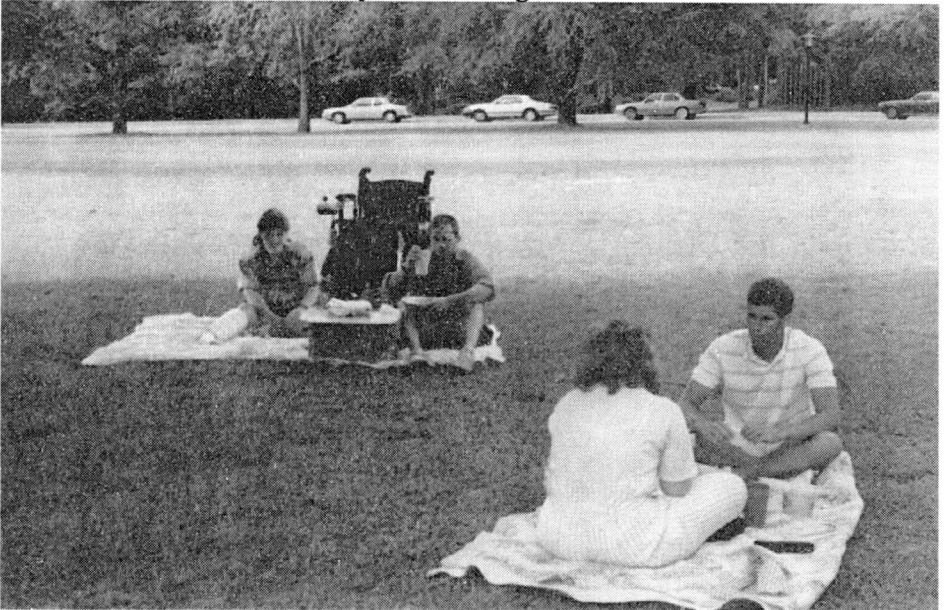
Melany and Charles on a picnic

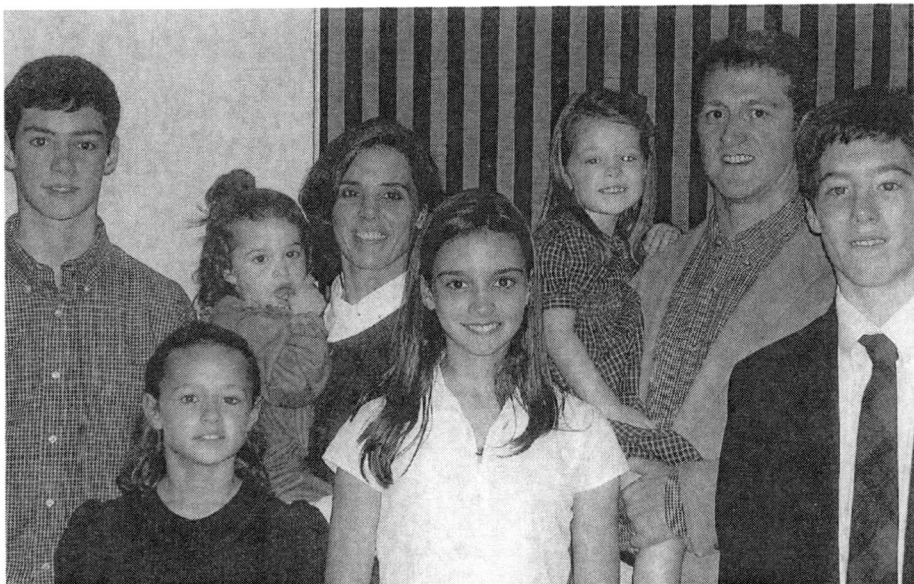

Noel and Jim Wilkerson and family

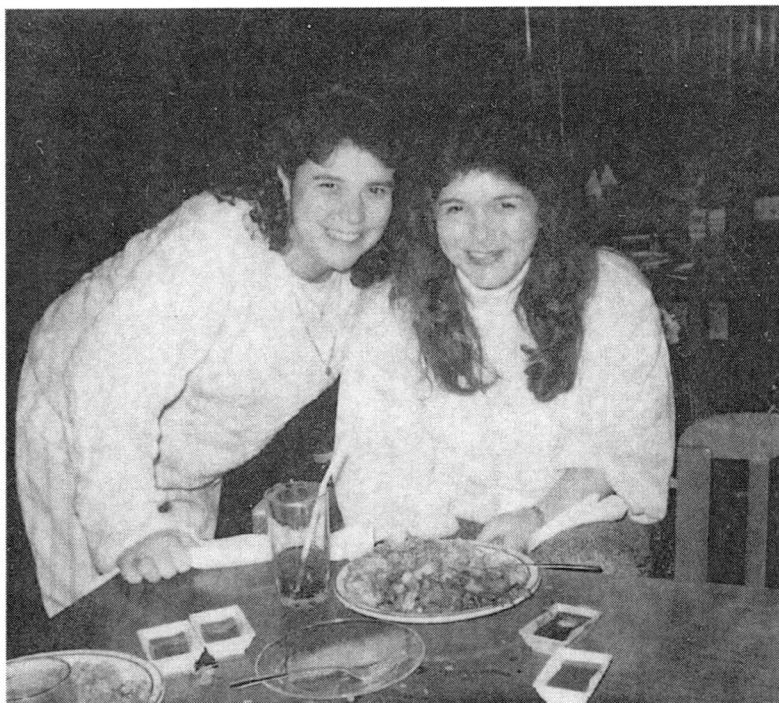

Rhonda and Melany

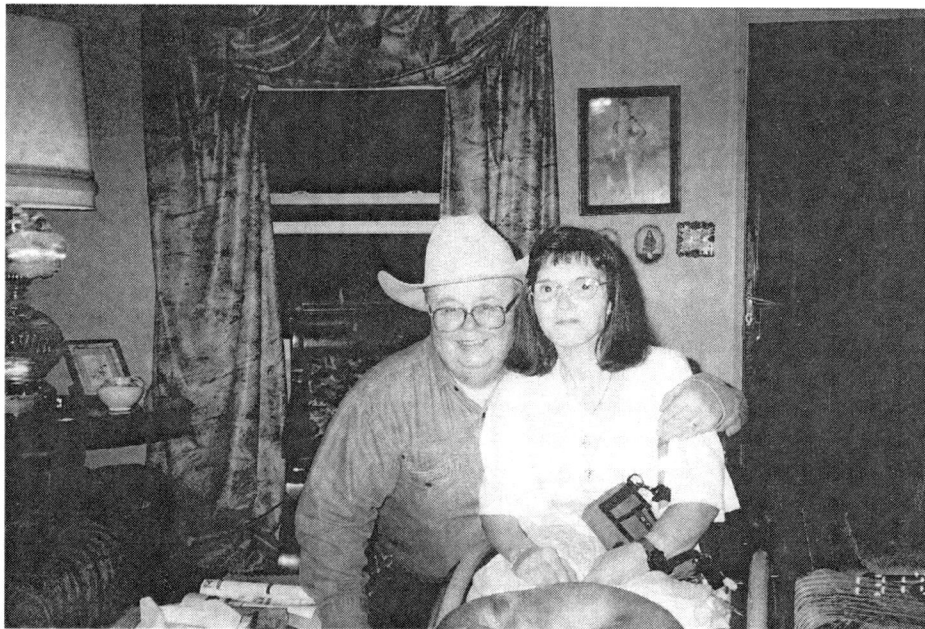

Robert Eubanks and Melany

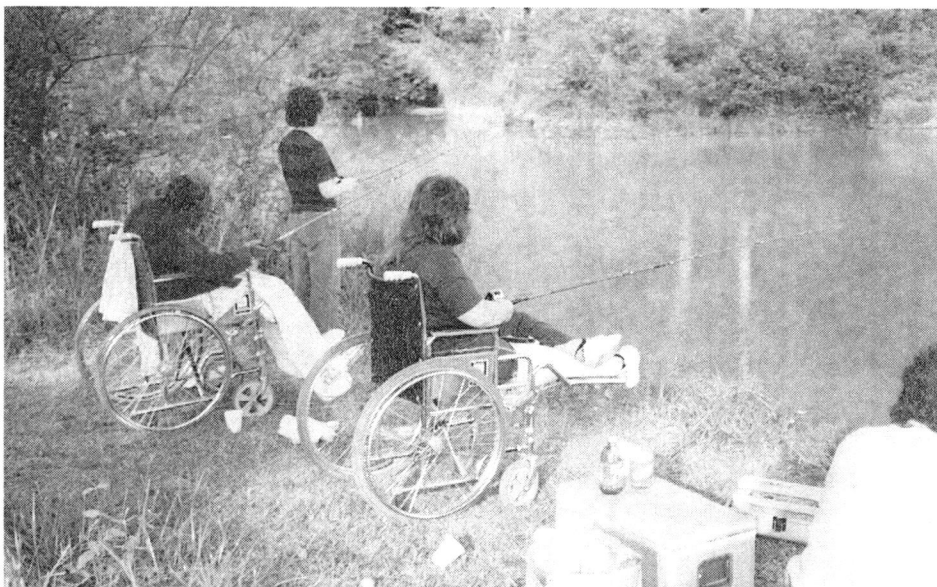

Melany fishing with friends from her internship

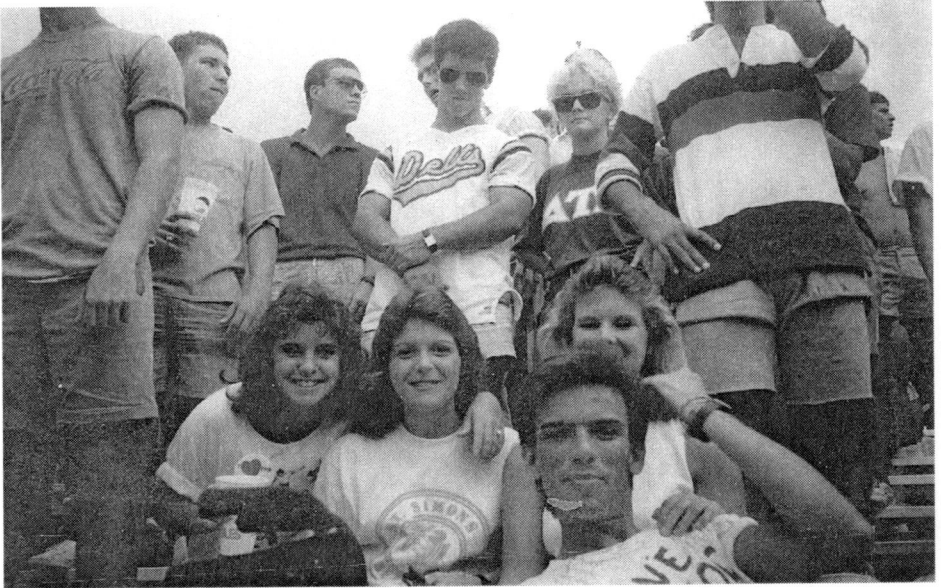
Melany with college friends at the beach

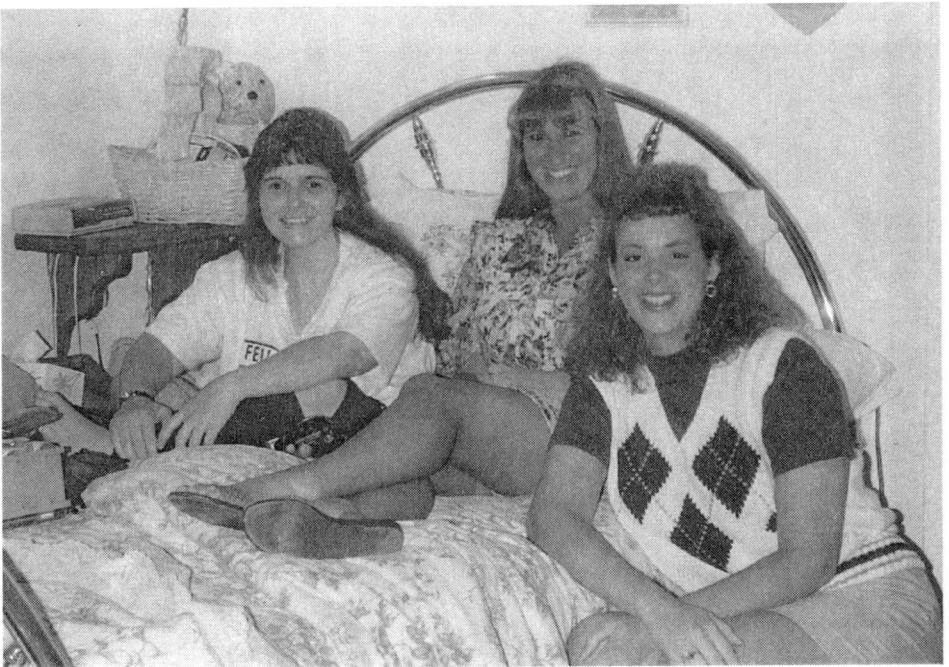
Melany, Lisa and Rebecca

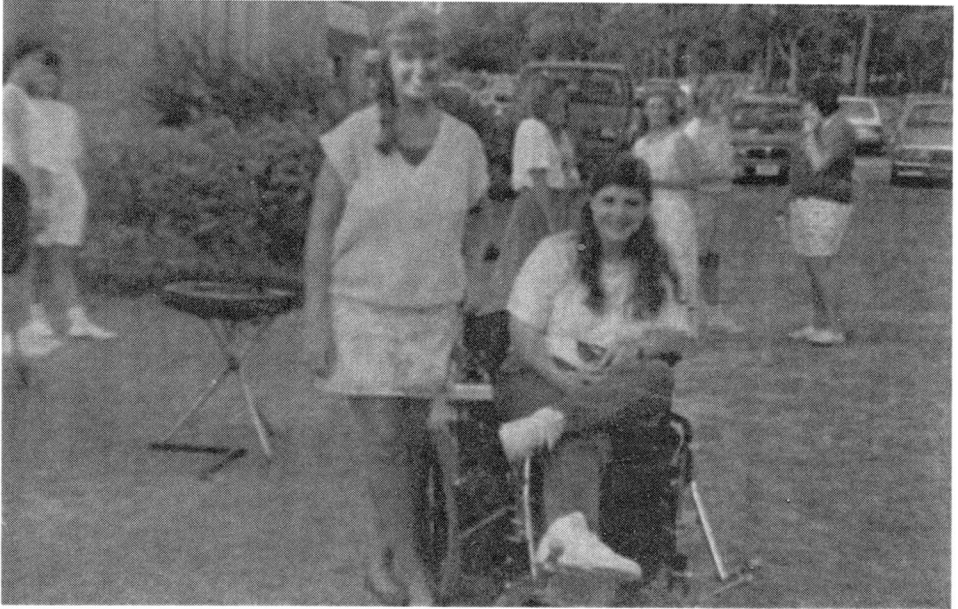

Lisa and Melany

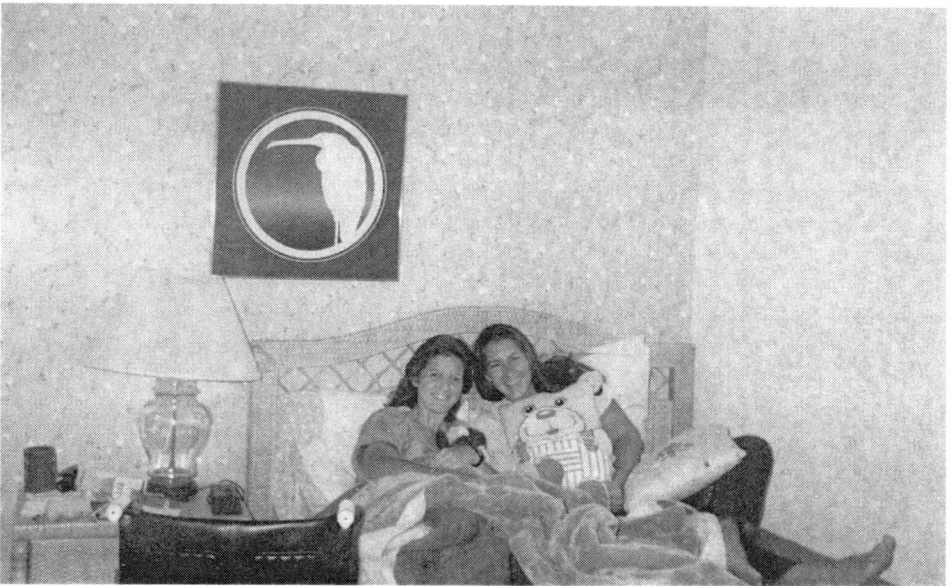

Melany and Julie

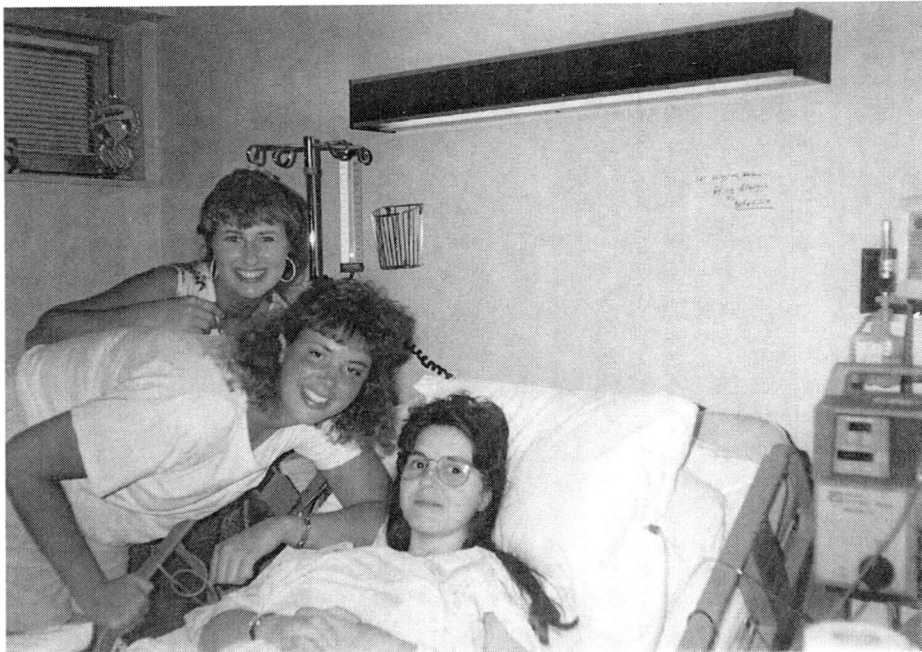

Lisa, Rebecca and Melany

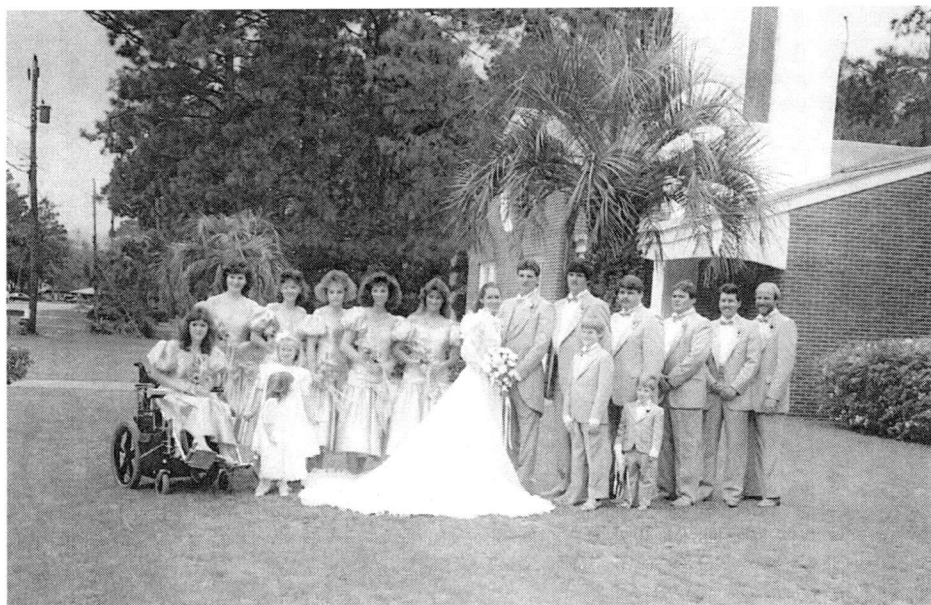

Melany in Julie and Ken Edwards' wedding

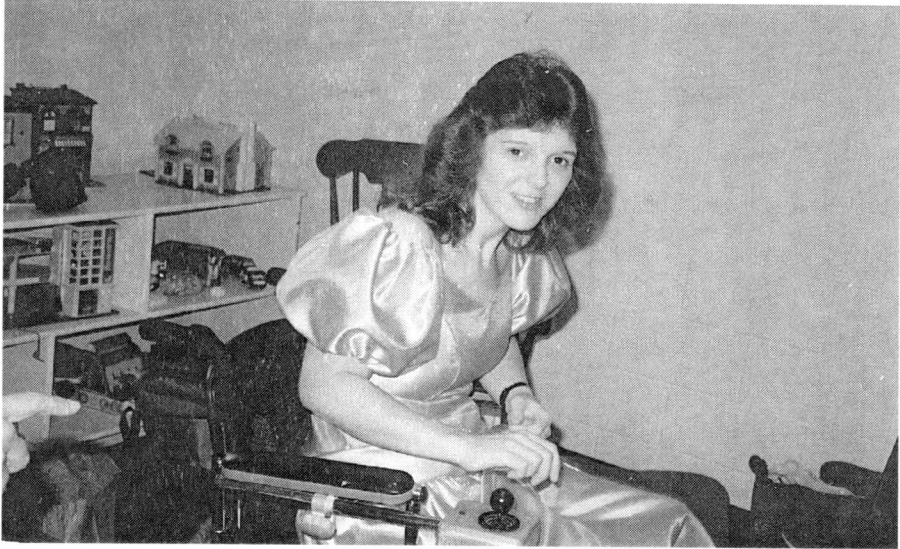
Melany as bridesmaid

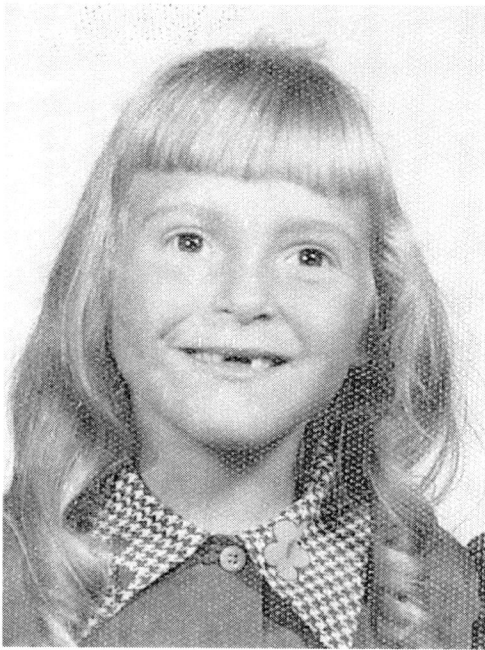
Melany at age 7 ("Snaggie")

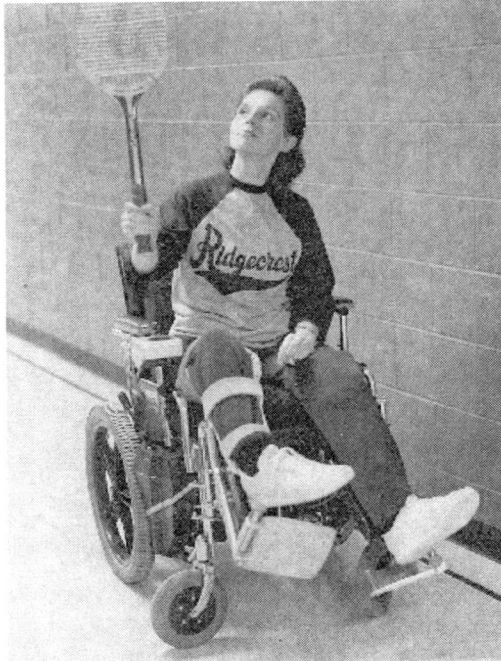
Melany playing badminton

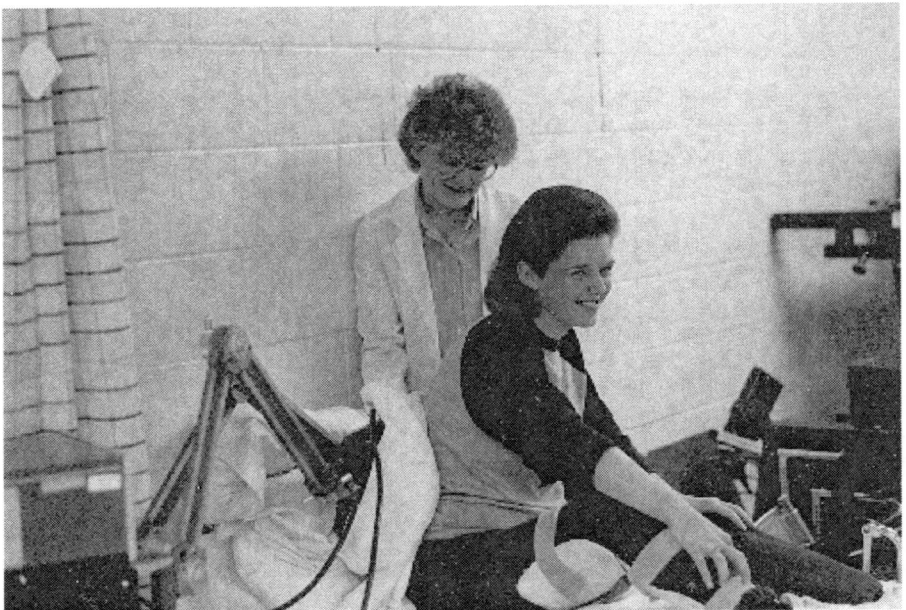
Melany with Physical Therapist Sally

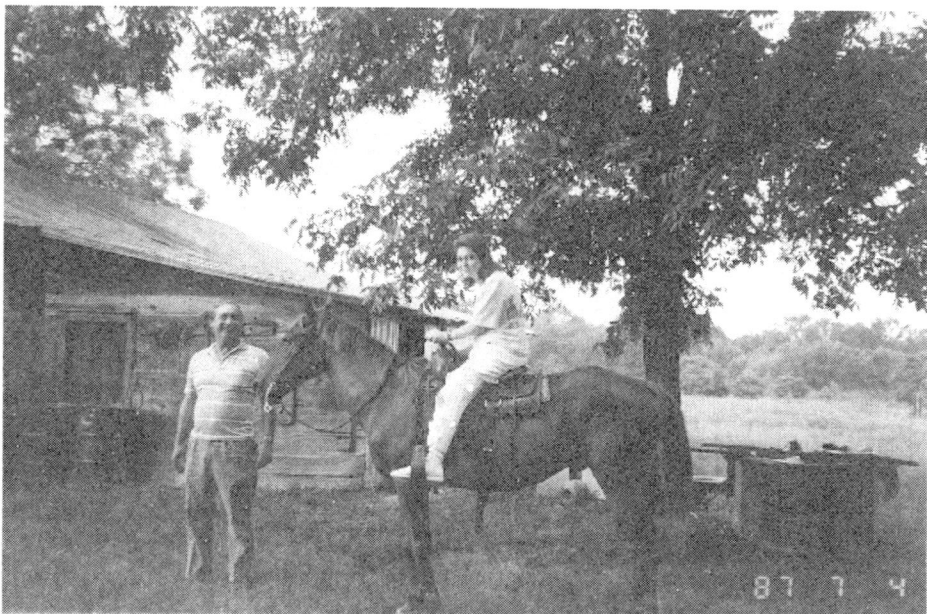

James with Melany on a horse

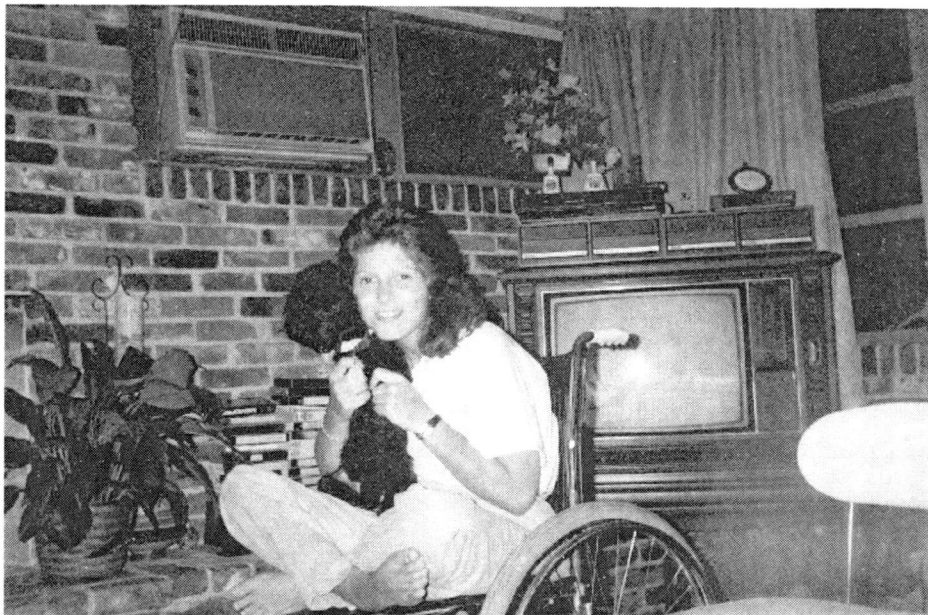

Melany and "Kooke"

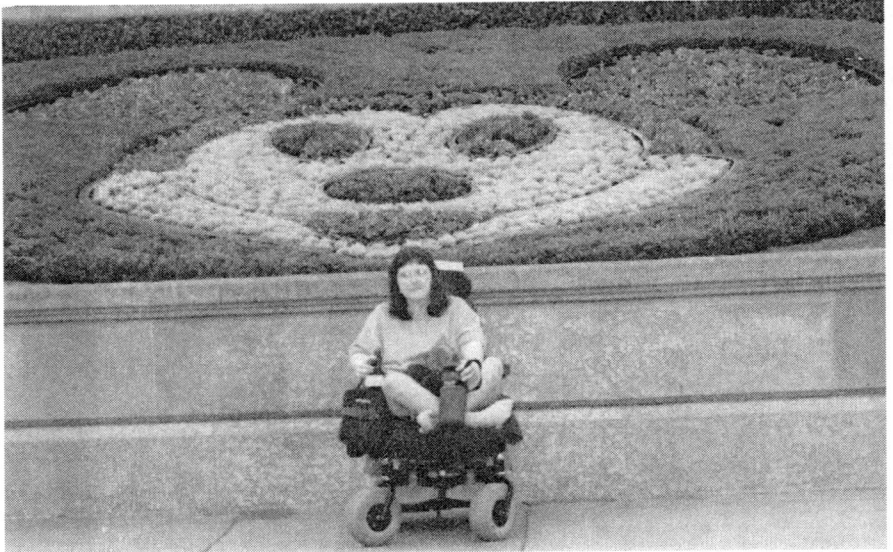

Melany at Disney

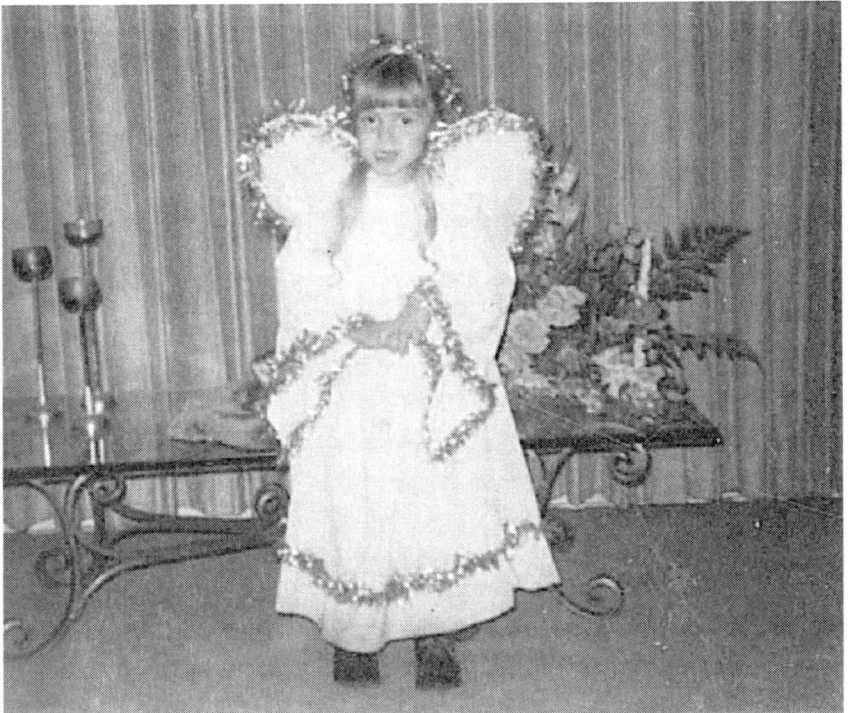

Melany as an angel on Halloween (age 5)

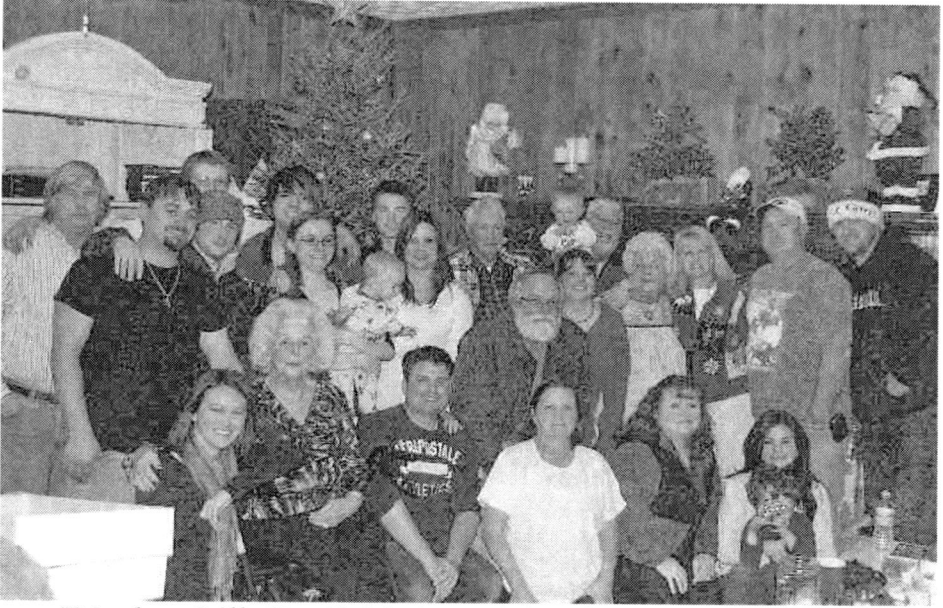

"My dear Stille Family" (minus eight who couldn't be there)

BIBLIOGRAPHY

Excerpts have been taken from the following sources in the production of this book:

Apples of Gold, compiled by Jo Petty, published by The C.R. Gibson Co., Norwalk, Connecticut

Parenting the Way God Parents by Katherine Koonce. Published by Multnomah Publishers, Sisters, Oregon.

Find Hope When Life is not Fair by Lee Ezell. Published by Revell, 2009.

Sitting by my Laughing Fire by Ruth Bell Graham. Published by Billy Graham Evangelistic Assocation, 2006, Charlotte, NC. Originally publsihed by Word Books, Waco, TX, 1977.

Streams in the Desert by Mrs. Charles E. Cowman. Published by Zondervan Publishing House (division of Harper-Collins), Grand, Rapids, MI. Copyright 1925 by Cowman Publications, renewed in 1953 and 1965. Copyright 1996 by Zondervan Publishing House.

CHAPTER & PAGE NOTES:

CHAPTER I--
1--Psalm 113:9 & Proverbs 15:13a
13--II Corinthians 12:9
20--Proverbs 22:6
21--II Chronicles 20:12
22--APPLES OF GOLD (p.25)
22--PARENTING THE WAY GOD PARENTS (p.185 & 207)

CHAPTER II--
23--I Peter 1:8b & Matt.19:13&14
28-29--Isaiah 45:11 & Proverbs 4:12 (Free translation)
35--PARENTING THE WAY GOD PARENTS (p.58 & 209)
35--APPLES OF GOLD (p.22)

CHAPTER III--
36--Hebrews 2:10 & Romans 8:18
51--II Corinthians 1:3&4 & II Corinthians 4:1
40--STREAMS IN THE DESERT (p.119)
54--FIND HOPE WHEN LIFE IS NOT FAIR (p.175)
54--PARENTING THE WAY GOD PARENTS (p.29)
54--STREAMS IN THE DESERT (301)

CHAPTER IV--
55--Isaiah 43:2 & Romans 8:26
55--Proverbs 22:15a
63--I Corinthians 2:14
64--STREAMS IN THE DESERT (p.19-20)
64--PARENTING THE WAY GOD PARENTS (p.155)

CHAPTER V--
65--Isaiah 7:11 & Luke 18:1
81--Nehemiah 8:10b
81--APPLES of GOLD (p. 20 & 31)

233--Ephesians 4:30
234-235--STREAMS IN THE DESERT (239)
236--FINDING HOPE WHEN LIFE IS NOT FAIR (P.118)
237--STREAMS IN THE DESERT (p.221)

CHAPTER XVII--
238--II Chronicles 14:11 (RV)
238--Psalm 46:10
241-242--http (Carol Adams)
249--STREAMS IN THE DESERT (281)
251--STREAMS IN THE DESERT (351)
251--STREAMS IN THE DESERT (106)
251--STREAMS IN THE DESERT (182)
252--http (Jo Lynn Jackson) --[Owner has copyright]
252--STREAMS IN THE DESERT (Bosch)
255--STREAMS IN THE DESERT (p.184)
257--STREAMS IN THE DESERT (p.294)
258--STREAMS IN THE DESERT (p.118)
258--STREAMS IN THE DESERT (p.27)

WANT ADDITIONAL COPIES OF THIS BOOK?

Additional copies of *Prittle, Prattle, Pain, Praise, Prayer, Peace and Perfection* are available wherever books are sold. If your local bookstore does not carry this book, ask the store to order it for you. You may also order online at Amazon.com or through other internet sellers, including the publisher at thomasmax.com. This book is also available in Kindle format for $4.99 from Amazon.com.

You may also order a *signed* copy directly from Nancy Wiggins. Please send your check or money order for $25 per copy (including postage and handling to addresses within the United States) to:

Nancy Wiggins
P.O. Box 16505
Augusta, GA 30919

As a bonus, you will receive, FREE, a DVD with each book ordered directly from the author. This DVD includes Melany's "Celebration of Life Service" from May 2008. You may also choose (from the DVD menu) to view only Melany's testimony given for a youth group at her church in 1998, 10 years before her death. These videos have been used in numerous church services to encourage people in helping and ministering to sick and disabled people. There is also a menu option for Nancy Wiggins' testimony of thanks to all at Melany's Celebration Service.

INSPIRATIONAL SPEAKING & SEMINARS

Nancy Wiggins is available for limited speaking and teaching engagements beginning in the fall of 2012 and throughout 2013, including, but not limited to:

SPEAKING TOPICS

1--Sovereignty of God
2--Prayer
3--Grief
4--Happiness and joy
5--Marriage and Remarriage
6--Managing Dreams for the Future

SEMINARS

Nancy is available to teach seminars on a variety of topics. If local (within 30 miles of Augusta), these will be presented in one hour segments weekly. Seminars out of the area can be done in one weekend, with flexible schedule according to church desires. Seminar topics include:

     1--Circle of Prayer (Six one hour sessions) -- In depth study of Prayer-How to really remember to pray for others.

     2--New Beginnings (Eight to ten hour sessions) for Singles/Singles Again . . . or anyone dealing with difficult issues including broken relationships, with family or friends.

     3--Grief (three--one hour sessions or two 90-minute sessions) for dealing with the death of a loved one, broken relationships or difficulties with adult children (often including remarriage of parent or child), financial or " just life" issues-- anything that causes us to grieve.

4--From Chaos to Calmness (three one hour sessions or two 90-minute sessions) -- How to survive problems or difficulties dealing with teenagers, and often adult children. Including drugs, alcohol abuse, rebellion, broken relationships.

Call or write for additional information and brochures (brochures available after October, 2012).

Nancy Merritt Wiggins
P.O. Box 16505
Augusta, Ga. 30919
E-mail: Wiggins.Nancy.inspiration@gmail.com

Phone: (706) 854-0949
Cell: (706) 830-8696

ABOUT THE AUTHOR

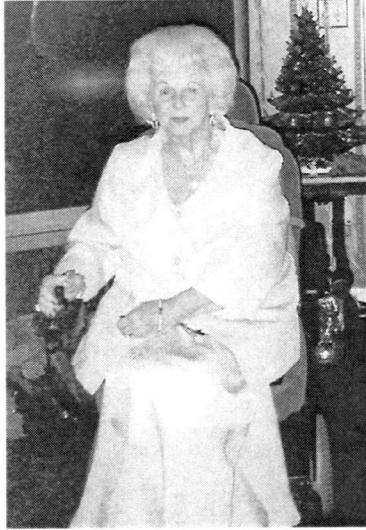

Nancy Wiggins was born in 1938 in Morgan, Georgia. She was born into a large, diverse, yet loving, family.

She married her high school sweetheart, James Wiggins, in 1955. They were active in the Curtis Baptist Church of Augusta, Ga . Nancy sang in the church choir and led the 5 year old Children's Choir for many years. She was WMU (Missions) Director for the church. She taught ten year old girls, and later the twelfth graders in Sunday School.

In 1980, she and James reorganized the Singles/Singles Again Sunday School Department. She wrote the lessons and material for this group. Later she followed with writing a manual, "Beginning Again" for Singles and others who had some disappointments in life. Those widowed, divorced or those dealing with broken relationships with family or friends. After writing several articles, she wrote a manual, "Circle of Prayer".

For years, until her daughter became very ill, she did three-day seminars on the manuals she wrote, as well as a Grief Recovery workshop. She also was a sought after speaker in churches, classes, banquets and Nursing Homes on "The Sovereignty of God," "Dreams," and "Christmas."

She and James had a wonderful life. The Lord blessed them with children. Their home was dedicated to the Lord. It was always open to welcome friends, their children's friends (regardless of how messy or loud they were), their grandson's friends and anyone who did not have a place to go for the Holidays.

The first child they had was stillborn on Christmas Eve, 1955. Their second child died at one year. The third child was killed in an automobile accident at age 37. Their last living child died at 41, after being confined to a wheelchair since age 12. All of the children brought much joy to their hearts and lives.

The family faced many difficulties of myriad diversities. Although their faith was tried and tested many times, they continued trusting the Lord. They did not allow situations or conditions to rob them of their joy in each other, their joy in life, or their joy in the Lord.

After being happily married for 53 years, James died in Feb. 2008 of lung cancer. Three months later in May, Melany was relieved of 30 years of pain and suffering as she joined her father and siblings in Heaven.

Since then, Nancy who had only desired to be a wife and mother found she was neither. She really did not know who she was. She had never lived alone, she did not know what to do. She started the arduous journey of widowhood, seeking to painfully walk through grief; praying to come out mentally, physically, emotionally and spiritually healthy.

ACKNOWLEDGMENTS AND THANKS

(1) **My Lord and Savior** for many years of sustaining grace and for me and my family. For allowing me to complete what Melany desired, the book to glorify His Name, to honor and thank the medical professionals, family, friends and all who faithfully prayed for her (and us) for over thirty-five years.

(2) **My Grandson, Jake** for helping me learn "Limited Computer Skills" so I could type the book. Also for being "On call" day or night to rescue me from my many mistakes. **Dr. Paul Joseph** also helped with the computer work.

(3) **Bobbie and Dick Moyer** for hours of reading, "critiquing," offering suggestions and correcting the manuscript.

(4) **Richard Magruder** for reading the entire manuscript, offering suggestions and encouraging me when I wanted to stop. For helping me with the medical terms, and for listening for hours to my ideas and ramblings.

(5) **My Stille Family, Tom, Darlene, Tim, Kimberly, James and Keith and their spouses** for the numerous ways they loved and helped me. Especially **Darlene** and **Josh** for copying hundreds of pages. And to **Keith** for helping me physically, financially and for supplying the videos.

(6) **Our church family at Curtis Baptist (Augusta), and at First Baptist (St. Simons Island)** and all church families that prayed for us so diligently, and sent cards and letters of encouragement.

(7) **All of my friends and family** for believing that I could complete this work. For all the prayers offered on my behalf.

(8) **All the employees of St. Joseph's Hospital (now Trinity)**. From the custodians, to all the staff, to the CEO for ALL

the many ways that they helped to care for Melany and the family through the years. Including the phone operators **Kitty** and **Tequilla** (sometimes our personal answering service [limited that is]).

(9) **Each one who wrote forewords and comments** and all the kind words that were said.

(10) **Stan Brassell** for the cover photo of Sunset at St. Simons Island.

(11) **Brad Kirkland and Josh Reid** for designing the cover of the book.

(12) Finally to **all the doctors** who worked so diligently and laboriously to try to help Melany through many health maladies and to help her to have the best quality of life possible. These include: **Dr. James Bennett, Dr. Zack Kilpatrick, Dr. Ted Everett, Dr. North Goodwin, Dr. Bill Barfield, Sr., Dr. Bill Barfield, Jr. Dr. William Welsh, Dr. Melvyn Haas, Dr. Charles McClure, Dr. Richard Magruder, Dr. Edward Crosland, Dr. Richard Sassnet, Dr. Mark Pitts, Dr. Harold Engler, Dr. Dennis Jones, Dr. Niti Carlson , Dr. Pomeroy Nichols, Dr. George Thurmond, Dr. John Kelley, Dr. Salim Oster, Dr. William Heery, Dr. Haroon Choudri, Dr. Michael Rivener, Dr. William Holden, Dr. Stanley Anderson, Dr. Joe Garrison, Dr. John Hudson, Dr. Jack Austin, Dr. Bradley Bertram and Dr. Carmel Joseph.**

CPSIA information can be obtained at www.ICGtesting.com
Printed in the USA
LVOW111201170612

286486LV00003B/3/P

9 780984 634774